对
初
学
者
的
七
十
個
中
医
要
方

SEVENTY ESSENTIAL

ESSENTIAL

TCM
Formulas
for
Beginners

BY

BOB FLAWS

BLUE POPPY PRESS

Published by:

BLUE POPPY PRESS
1775 LINDEN AVE.
BOULDER, CO 80304

FIRST EDITION, SEPTEMBER 1994

ISBN 0-936185-59-7 LC #94-77987

The information in this book is given in good faith. However, the translators and the publisher cannot be held responsible for any error or omission. Nor can they be held in any way responsible for treatment given on the basis of information contained in this book. The publisher make this information available to English language readers for scholarly and research purposes only.

The publishers do not advocate nor endorse self-medication by laypersons. Chinese medicine is a professional medicine. Laypersons interested in availing themselves of the treatments described in this book should seek out a qualified professional practitioner of Chinese medicine.

COMP Designation: Original work and functionally translated compilation

Printed at Westview Press, Boulder, CO on acid free, recycled paper.
Cover printed at C & M Press, Denver, CO
Cover calligraphy by Michael Sullivan (Seiho)
Other calligraphies provided by Samuel Chang of Qualiherb, Inc.

10 9 8 7 6 5 4 3 2

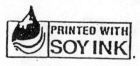

recycled paper

PRINTED WITH SOY INK

Acknowledgement

The calligraphies that grace this book are all traditional mnemonic verses for memorizing the name, ingredients, and major use of the most important standard TCM medicinal formulas. They have been commissioned and provided by Samuel Chang of Qualiherb, Inc. The author and publishers are very grateful for this beautiful contribution.

Preface

This book is a basic repertoire of 70 Chinese herbal formulas. At Traditional Chinese Medicine (TCM) colleges in the People's Republic of China, undergraduates in the internal medicine division are taught a basic repertoire of between 50 and 100 formulas in a course called *fang ji xue*. Literally, this means the study of formulas and prescriptions. In this course, students are taught and are expected to memorize one or two formulas from each of the 21 major categories of herbal formulas. Since some of these major categories are comprised of two or more subcategories, the total number of formulas memorized comes up to approximately four score.

In the Chinese TCM literature, there are three types of books containing collections of herbal formulas. These are *fang ji xue* textbooks, clinical manuals on the treatment of modern TCM's various specialties, and formula compendia books. However, it is important that beginners in the study of TCM formulas and prescriptions start with a *fang ji xue* text as opposed to a less structured formula compendium. This is because such *fang ji xue* texts as this help to clarify and instil the TCM methodology beyond just being a repository of numerous formulas.

Modern TCM bases its treatment on a very specific, rational, step by step methodology. In Chinese, this is called *bian zheng lun zhi*, basing treatment on a discrimination of patterns. When a TCM practitioner is presented with a patient with high blood pressure, their first job is to discriminate this patient's TCM pattern. This pattern is the professionally agreed upon description of the entirety of the patient's signs and symptoms as opposed to simply those symptoms pathognomonic of their disease. Such patterns in hypertensive patients may include liver yang hyperactivity; liver/kidney yin vacuity; yin and yang dual vacuity; loss of balance of the *chong* and *ren*; harbored wind; harbored phlegm; and harbored stasis. Depending upon which pattern their patient exhibits, the practitioner is guided to a certain category of formulas via their statement of treatment principles.

For instance, if the patient's pattern is liver yang hyperactivity, the treatment principles are to level the liver and drain fire. Thus the practitioner knows that they should choose a formula from the heavy settling spirit-calming category of formulas. In addition, they need to find a formula within that category which levels the liver specifically and drains fire. If the patient's pattern is liver/kidney yin vacuity, then the treatment principles are to nourish yin and boost the kidneys. This means the practitioner will find their guiding formula in the supplementing category of formulas, subcategory supplementing yin. If the patient's pattern is yin and yang dual vacuity, the treatment principles are to invigorate yang and enrich yin. In this case, the guiding formula will be found under the supplementing category, subcategory supplementing yang. If the patient's pattern is loss of regularity between the *chong* and *ren*, then the treatment principles are to warm and enrich while using bitter to also drain. Although this is not immediately apparent from the English words used, the practitioner will also find their guiding formula under the yang-supplementing prescriptions. Likewise, if there is harbored wind, this wind should be extinguished and the formula will be found under formulas which treat wind. If there is harbored phlegm, the principle is to transform phlegm and the formula will be found under the phlegm-transforming category. This then needs to be further divided into hot phlegm and damp phlegm subcategories. And if there is harbored stasis, the principles are to quicken the blood and transform stasis. In this case, the appropriate guiding formula will be found under the blood-rectifying category, blood-quickening, stasis-transforming subcategory.

In other words, according to TCM *bian zheng lun zhi* methodology, one first establishes the TCM pattern discrimination or diagnosis. Based on this, one states the treatment principles necessary to rectify the imbalance inherent in the name of the pattern. Usually there will be more than a single principle. For example, for liver depression, qi stagnation, the principles are to course the liver, resolve depression, and rectify the qi. One of the 21 categories of formulas is the *li qi ji* or qi-rectifying formulas. Therefore, based on these principles, one should choose a formula from the *li qi ji* group of prescriptions.

Once one has identified the proper category of prescriptions, one then looks through the formulas listed under that category to find one that is empirically known to treat the specific patient's major complaint and their idiosyncratic signs and symptoms. For instance, under the clearing heat from the viscera and bowels category, there are formulas for the liver, lungs, heart, gallbladder, stomach, intestines, etc. For heat in the heart, one should choose a formula that is designed to clear heat from specifically that organ. Further, certain formulas are known through long clinical practice to treat certain diseases or signs and symptoms. If the patient's disease diagnosis is vertigo and their TCM pattern diagnosis is internal stirring of phlegm mixed with dampness, one not only should choose a formula from the *zhi feng ji* or wind-treating category of formulas but also one that is known to treat vertigo.

In *How to Write a TCM Herbal Formula*, I have written about this step by step progression from pattern diagnosis to treatment principles to category of formula to specific formula in greater detail. In this book I am primarily interested in presenting a basic repertoire of formulas divided according to a slightly pared down version of these traditional categories of prescriptions. I have deliberately tried to keep the number of formulas given in this book as few as possible. This list of formulas is almost identical to the one my own TCM herbal medicine teacher, Dr. Chen Wei, taught me at the Shanghai College of Traditional Chinese Medicine. If one learns and understands how to modify this core group of formulas with additions and subtractions, one will have a basic repertoire of formulas for most clinical occasions. One will then also be able to learn and understand other formulas in the same categories more easily, since one will understand the principles of formula-writing and medicinal synergy at work in the key representative formula in each category.

This book is not meant to either replace or compete with Bensky & Barolet's *Chinese Herbal Medicine: Formulas & Strategies.* That book should be every TCM internal medicine student's bible. It likewise is a *fang ji xue* text. It is a great reference and should sit on the desk of every English-speaking practitioner of TCM internal medicine. For more detailed information on all the formulas discussed herein, the reader is referred to that text. However, because of its size and comprehensiveness, it is not the easiest book for students to carry around and study from. This book, on the other hand, is meant as a bare-bones skeleton or outline for prioritized study by undergraduates and neophytes.

It should be mentioned that before studying formulas and prescriptions, one should first have completed a course known in Chinese as *ben cao xue*, the study of the materia medica. It is impossible to understand formulas and the logic of their composition if one does not know the nature (*i.e.* temperature), flavor, channel enterings, functions, indications, contraindications and prohibitions, dosages, and combinations of a basic repertoire of between 3-400 Chinese medicinals. Readers who do not yet have such a basic understanding of individual TCM medicinals should first take up that study before attempting to use this book.

The order of this book and the names of the categories of formulas are based on the Shanghai Science & Technology Press' *Fang Ji Xue (The Study of Formulas & Prescriptions)*, 1986 edition. The material in this book is based on that book and other Chinese formula compendia texts, Dr. Chen's lecture notes, several English language texts listed in the bibliography, and my own experience and research.

It is not a translation of the Shanghai Science & Technology Press'
Fang Ji Xue but is rather an original creation based on a number of
sources. In trying to keep the number of formulas to an absolute
minimum, I have not discussed nor given representative formulas for
some of the categories discussed in *Fang Ji Xue*. The treatment of
these conditions, such as vomiting and ulcers, is discussed under
formula additions and subtractions under other categories and
formulas.

I have used Nigel Wiseman's translational terminology for technical
terms throughout as found in his and Ken Boss' *Glossary of Chinese
Medical Terms and Acupuncture Points*. As I have mentioned in
numerous other prefaces, the understanding of TCM as a self-contained
system of thought and practice is largely based on the logic inherent
in the Chinese language. Therefore, it is imperative that student's TCM
vocabulary be as technically precise, accurate, and as close to the
Chinese as possible.

Under indications for each formula, I first give the TCM pattern or
zheng. Following this and separated by a period are a list of Western
medical diseases and conditions. The reader should take care that only
those with the *zheng* under discussion should be treated with that
particular formula. In my experience, it is extremely important to base
treatment on a combination of TCM *bian zheng* diagnosis and a disease
diagnosis, be it modern Western or traditional Chinese. Practitioners
should not attempt to apply these formulas based on Western disease
categories alone.

Bob Flaws
July 1994

补中益气术陈

升柴参草当归耆

劳役内伤功独擅

点注汤君外试曰

木鱼苓术易汤术

调中益气畅脾神

Mnemonic verse for learning *Bu Zhong Yi Qi Tang*

Contents

1

Jie Biao Ji
Exterior-relieving Formulas

Generally speaking, exterior-relieving formulas include medicinals which can relieve or resolve exterior patterns. Typically, they expel external evils by promoting mild sweating. This diaphoresis out-thrusts and expels the pathogens. In addition, they resolve the muscles and promote the eruption of rashes or pox. They may also be used for the treatment of sores in the exterior and recent onset edema if either are accompanied by aversion to cold, fever, and other exterior pattern signs and symptoms. Exterior patterns are due to external invasion of the six environmental excesses. These include wind, cold, summerheat, dampness, dryness, and fire. The distinguishing characteristics of an exterior pattern are aversion to cold and wind, fever, headache, muscular aches and pains, and a floating pulse.

There are two main types of exterior patterns: hot and cold. Because the causative factors and the body's reaction to disease is different, these two types of exterior patterns require treatment with different medicinals. In exterior cold patterns, aversion to cold is pronounced, there is slight fever, no particular thirst, either no sore throat or just a tickle in the throat, a clear nasal discharge, a floating, tight pulse, and a thin, white tongue coating. In an exterior heat pattern, there is less aversion to cold and wind, more extreme fever, definite thirst, definite sore throat, yellow, sticky nasal mucus, a floating, rapid pulse, and a red tongue tip with a yellow coating. Based on these two main types of exterior patterns, exterior-relieving formulas are divided into two main subcategories: 1) acrid, warm, exterior-relieving formulas and 2) acrid, cool, exterior-relieving formulas.

There is, however, a third category of exterior-relieving formulas. These are called supporting the righteous and relieving the exterior formulas. They are used when the body is vacuous but has been invaded by external evils manifesting as exterior patterns. In this case, it is still necessary to relieve the exterior. However, because the righteous is vacuous, one must use medicinals which supplement and boost (qi) and assist yang combined with exterior-relieving medicinals. These types of formulas are good for the treatment of children whose source qi is not full. They can also be used on postpartum women or after major disease when there is bodily vacuity and weakness and invasion of wind, cold, damp evils manifesting as an exterior pattern.

Method of Preparation & Administration:

Acrid medicinals are light and windy in nature and easily spread outward and upward. Therefore, they should not be cooked for lengthy periods as this will disperse their therapeutic effect. They should only be decocted for from 20-30 minutes maximum. Once the water is boiling, decoct for a further 5-10 minutes with a large fire (*i.e.*, high heat). Exterior-relieving medicinals should be taken while still warm and away from cold and drafts. The patient should be instructed to put on more clothes.

Cautions in Using Exterior-relieving Medicinals:

The right degree of perspiration induced by exterior-relieving medicinals is a mild perspiration over the entire body. If perspiration is too much, righteous qi will be damaged. This is especially so in children and the aged. Excessive perspiration will also damage fluids and humors.

Patients may exhibit both exterior and interior patterns. In such cases, first relieve the exterior and then treat the interior. However, if both exterior and interior are affected to the same degree, treat both simultaneously.

The Five Contraindications of Exterior-relieving Formulas:

1. Do not relieve the exterior once exterior patterns have transmuted into interior patterns.
2. Do not relieve the exterior once pox and rashes have erupted.
3. Do not relieve the exterior once sores have ulcerated.
4. Do not relieve the exterior for the treatment of edema due to vacuity.
5. Do not relieve the exterior if there is dehydration due to vomiting and diarrhea.

1.1 *Xin Wen Jie Biao Ji* (Acrid, warm, exterior-relieving formulas)

Representative formulas:

A. *Ma Huang Tang* (Ephedra Decoction)

Composition:

Herba Ephedrae (*Ma Huang*), remove the joints, 6g
Ramulus Cinnamomi (*Gui Zhi*), 4g
Semen Pruni Armeniacae (*Xing Ren*), remove the skin and tips, 9g
Radix Glycyrrhizae (*Gan Cao*), mix-fried, 3g

Functions: Emits perspiration and relieves the exterior, diffuses the lungs and levels wheezing

Indications: External invasion, wind cold. Common cold, cough, asthma, typhoid fever, pneumonia, bronchitis, measles, rhinitis, stuffy nose, neurosis, nocturnal enuresis, cystitis, and rheumatoid arthritis.

Main signs & symptoms: Aversion to cold, fever, headache, body aches, absence of sweat, possible wheezing, a thin, white tongue coating, and a rapid, tight pulse

Formula explanation:

Ephedra is bitter, acrid, and warm and enters the lung channel. It is capable of emitting and overpassing the yang qi of the body. It thus emits perspiration and relieves the exterior, diffuses the lungs and levels wheezing. Therefore, it is the sovereign medicinal in this formula. It is aided by Cinnamon, its minister, which strengthens its effect of inducing perspiration at the same time as the Cinnamon warms the channels and scatters cold. Thus the constructive is no longer astringed and the defensive is no longer depressed. Armeniaca, the assistant, helps Ephedra level wheezing while it diffuses the lungs and expels evil. Mix-fried Licorice regulates and harmonizes the diffusing and downbearing of Ephedra and, along with Armeniaca, relaxes and moderates Ephedra. Thus righteous qi is not consumed and damaged.

Additions & subtractions:

If there is no aversion to cold, subtract Cinnamon and add raw Rhizoma Zingiberis (*Sheng Jiang*). This results in the formation of *San Ao Tang* (Three Unbindings Decoction).

If there is wheezing, cough with copious, clear, white phlegm but only mild fever, chills, bodily aching, and headache, subtract Cinnamon and add Radix Peucedani (*Qian Hu*).

4

If there is cough and excessive phlegm, subtract Cinnamon and add Cortex Radicis Mori (*Sang Bai Pi*), Fructus Perillae Frutescentis (*Zi Su Zi*), Sclerotium Rubrum Poriae Cocos (*Chi Fu Ling*), and Pericarpium Citri Reticulatae (*Chen Pi*). This results in *Hua Gai San* (Florid Canopy Powder).

For wheezing, chest oppression, and coughing of white, watery phlegm, add Fructus Perillae Frutescentis (*Su Zi*) and Pericarpium Citri Reticulatae (*Chen Pi*).

For lung heat patterns, subtract Cinnamon and add Gypsum (*Shi Gao*). This results in *Ma Xing Gan Shi Tang* (Ephedra, Armeniaca, Licorice, & Gypsum Decoction).

If there is exterior cold/interior heat, simply add Gypsum (*Shi Gao*).

If there is simultaneous qi vacuity, add Radix Astragali Membranacei (*Huang Qi*).

If there is sore throat, reduce the Cinnamon by half and add Radix Trichosanthis Kirlowii (*Tian Hua Fen*) and Rhizoma Belamcandae (*She Gan*).

In the initial stage of *bi* syndrome, if there is runny nose, edema, or dysuria, add Rhizoma Atractylodis Macrocephalae (*Bai Zhu*). This results in *Ma Huang Jia Zhu Tang* (Ephedra with Atractylodis Added Decoction).

For wind damp muscular *bi* and joint pain, add Semen Lachryma-jobi (*Yi Yi Ren*). This results in *Ma Xing Yi Gan Tang* (Ephedra, Armeniaca, Coix, & Licorice Decoction).

For severe arthritis, add Rhizoma Atractylodis (*Cang Zhu*), Radix Gentianae Macrophyllae (*Qin Jiao*), and Ramus Lonicerae Japonicae (*Ren Dong Teng*).

For high fever and thirst indicating the constructive has been damaged, add Gypsum (*Shi Gao*), raw Rhizoma Zingiberis (*Sheng Jiang*), and Fructus Zizyphi Jujubae (*Da Zao*). This results in *Da Qing Long Tang* (Large Blue-green Dragon Decoction).

B. *Gui Zhi Tang* (Cinnamon Twig Decoction)

Composition:

Ramulus Cinnamomi (*Gui Zhi*), 9g
Radix Paeoniae Lactiflorae (*Shao Yao*), 9g
Radix Glycyrrhizae (*Gan Cao*), mix-fried, 6g
raw Rhizoma Zingiberis (*Sheng Jiang*), 9g
Fructus Zizyphi Jujubae (*Da Zao*), 12 pieces

Method of administration: Traditionally it is advised that one eat rice soup after taking this decoction in order to promote perspiration.

Functions: Relieves the muscles and emits the exterior, regulates and harmonizes the constructive and defensive

Indications: 1) External invasion, wind cold in cases of exterior vacuity of the *tai yang*; 2) internal diseases with loss of harmony between the constructive and defensive, such as after prolonged disease or postpartum. Common cold, neuralgia, headache, abdominal pain due to chills, bodily weakness and vacuity, eclampsia, and neurasthenia.

Main signs & symptoms: 1) Exterior vacuity: sweating but yet continuing aversion to wind and fever, stiff neck, stuffy nose, no thirst, no sore throat, a thin, white, moist tongue coating, and a floating, relaxed/retarded or floating, weak pulse. 2) Internal disease with loss of harmony between the constructive and defensive: intermittent aversion to heat and cold, aversion to wind, plus sweating.

Contraindications:

1. Exterior repletion patterns of the *tai yang*
2. Hemorrhagic conditions
3. A red tongue with a yellow or peeled coating

Formula explanation:

In this case, there is wind cold in the exterior. However, there is also exterior vacuity, the striae (*cou li*) are not secure, and the defensive is strong and the constructive is weak. Therefore, Cinnamon is used as the sovereign in order to resolve the muscles, emit the exterior, and scatter externally invading wind cold. Peony as the minister medicinal boosts yin and restrains the constructive. When Cinnamon and Peony are combined together, one treats a strong defensive and the other a weak constructive, thus regulating and harmonizing constructive and defensive. Fresh Ginger is acrid and warm. It helps Cinnamon relieve the muscles and is also able to warm the stomach and stop vomiting. Red Dates are sweet and neutral and help boost the qi and supplement the center. They are also able to enrich the spleen and engender fluids. Red Dates and Ginger combined together make room in the spleen and stomach for the generation and emission of qi and regulate and harmonize the constructive and defensive. Likewise, Red Dates assist Peony in harmonizing the constructive and defensive. Mix-fried Licorice is used for two reasons. First, it boosts the qi and harmonizes the center. Together with Cinnamon, it resolves the muscles, and together with Peony, it boosts yin. Secondly, it regulates and harmonizes all the other medicinals.

Additions & subtractions:

For marked stuffy nose and sneezing, add Radix Ledebouriellae Sesloidis (*Fang Feng*) and Flos Magnoliae (*Xin Yi*).

For shortness of breath and rough breathing, add Cortex Magnoliae Officinalis (*Hou Po*) and Semen Pruni Armeniacae (*Xing Ren*). This results in *Gui Zhi Jia Hou Po Xing Ren Tang* (Cinnamon, Magnolia, & Armeniaca Decoction).

For distention and heaviness in the head, add Flos Chrysanthemi Morifolii (*Ju Hua*) and Periostracum Cicadae (*Chan Tui*).

If there is excessive sweating, increase the dosage of Peony and decrease by one-third the dosages of Cinnamon, Ginger, and Licorice. Then add Radix Astragali Membranacei (*Huang Qi*) and Radix Ledebouriellae Sesloidis (*Fang Feng*).

For severe headache, substitute Radix Rubrus Paeoniae Lactiflorae (*Chi Shao*) for White Peony and add Radix Et Rhizoma Ligustici (*Gao Ben*).

For severe vomiting, increase the dosages of Peony and Ginger and add Pericarpium Citri Reticulatae (*Chen Pi*) and Cortex Magnoliae Officinalis (*Hou Po*).

If there is wind, cold, damp *bi*, add Rhizoma Curcumae Longae (*Jiang Huang*), Herba Cum Radice Asari (*Xi Xin*), and Radix Clematidis (*Wei Ling Xian*).

For stiff neck and shoulder, add Radix Puerariae Lobatae (*Ge Gen*). This results in *Gui Zhi Jia Ge Gen Tang* (Cinnamon & Pueraria Decoction).

If there is slippery essence, excessive dreams, frigid lower extremities, dizziness, and hair loss, add Os Draconis (*Long Gu*) and Concha Ostreae (*Mu Li*). This results in *Gui Zhi Jia Long Gu Mu Li Tang* (Cinnamon, Dragon Bone, & Oyster Shell Decoction).

If there is external invasion of wind cold with simultaneous spleen/kidney dual vacuity, add Herba Ephedra (*Ma Huang*), Rhizoma Atractylodis Macrocephalae (*Bai Zhu*), Rhizoma Anemarrhenae (*Zhi Mu*), Radix Praeparatus Aconiti Carmichaeli (*Fu Zi*), and Radix Ledebouriellae Sesloidis (*Fang Feng*) and change fresh Ginger to dry Rhizoma Zingiberis (*Gan Jiang*). This results in *Gui Zhi Shao Yao Zhi Mu Tang* (Cinnamon, Peony, & Anemarrhena Decoction). This treats wind damp joint pain, atony of the lower extremities, difficulty breathing, and paralysis.

If there is blood vacuity with the above pattern, to *Gui Zhi Shao Yao Zhi Mu Tang* add Radix Angelicae Sinensis (*Dang Gui*), Rhizoma Ligustici Wallichii (*Chuan Xiong*), prepared Radix Rehmanniae (*Shu Di*), Radix Astragali Membranacei (*Huang Qi*), and Sclerotium Poriae Cocos (*Fu Ling*).

For paralysis and palsy, to *Gui Zhi Shao Yao Zhi Mu Tang* add Radix Stephaniae Tetrandrae (*Han Fan Ji*), Radix Panacis Ginseng (*Ren Shen*), Radix Scutellariae Baicalensis (*Huang Qin*), Rhizoma Ligustici Wallichii (*Chuan Xiong*), and Semen Pruni Armeniacae (*Xing Ren*). This results in *Xiao Shu Ming Tang* (Minor Accept Destiny Decoction) with Atractylodis Macrocephalae and Anemarrhena.

And for arthritis of the upper extremities, to *Gui Zhi Shao Yao Zhi Mu Tang* add Radix Et Rhizoma Notopterygii (*Qiang Huo*), Herba Cum Radice Asari (*Xi Xin*), Radix Stephaniae Tetrandrae (*Han Fang Ji*), and Sclerotium Poriae Cocos (*Fu Ling*). This results in *Ma Huang Qiang Huo Tang* (Ephedra & Notopterygium Decoction) with Anemarrhena, Peony, and Aconite added.

1.2 *Xin Liang Jie Biao Ji* (Acrid, cool, exterior-relieving formulas)

Representative formulas:

A. *Sang Ju Yin* (Morus & Chrysanthemum Drink)

Composition:

Folium Mori Albi (*Sang Ye*), 7.5g
Flos Chrysanthemi Morifolii (*Ju Hua*), 3g
Semen Pruni Armeniacae (*Xing Ren*), 6g
Fructus Forsythiae Suspensae (*Lian Qiao*), 5g
Herba Menthae (*Bo He*), 2.5g
Radix Platycodi Grandiflori (*Jie Geng*), 6g
Radix Glycyrrhizae (*Gan Cao*), 2.5g, raw
Rhizoma Phragmitis Communis (*Lu Gen*), 6g

Functions: To course wind and clear heat, diffuse the lungs and stop cough

Indications: Wind heat, initial stage. Common cold, flus, acute bronchitis, acute tonsillitis, epidemic conjunctivitis, headache, vertigo, acute tracheitis.

Main signs & symptoms: Cough, fever, a red, sore throat, slight fever, a thin, white or slightly yellow tongue coating with a red tongue proper, and a floating, rapid pulse

Formula explanation:

In this formula, Folium Mori and Chrysanthemum are the sovereign medicinals. Morus penetrates and clears heat from the network vessels of the lungs. Chrysanthemum clears and scatters wind heat in the upper burner. Mint, acrid and cool, is the minister medicinal. It assists Morus and Chrysanthemum scatter upper burner wind heat. Among Platycodon and Armeniaca, one upbears and one downbears, thus resolving the muscles, depurating the lungs, and, therefore, stopping coughing. Forsythia clears heat above the diaphragm. Phragmites clears heat, engenders fluids, and stops thirst. These two are the assistant medicinals. Licorice regulates and harmonizes these medicinals and is the messenger medicinal. The combination of Licorice and Platycodon is called *Gan Cao Jie Geng Tang* (Licorice & Platycodon Decoction). This is especially for patients with cough and phlegm which is difficult to expectorate accompanied by a slight tickling sensation in the throat. Combined, these medicinals have the function of coursing wind and clearing heat, diffusing the lungs and stopping cough.

Additions & subtractions:

If there is heat in the qi division manifesting as severe cough and thirst, add Gypsum (*Shi Gao*) and Rhizoma Anemarrhenae (*Zhi Mu*).

If lung heat is serious and is causing coughing, add Radix Scutellariae Baicalensis (*Huang Qin*) to clear heat and stop coughing.

If there is thirst, add Radix Trichosanthis Kirlowii (*Tian Hua Fen*) to clear heat and engender fluids. If lung heat cough is serious and has damaged the network vessels causing coughing up of bloody mucus, add Rhizoma Imperatae Cylindricae (*Mao Gen*), Nodus Nelumbinis Nuciferae (*Ou Jie*), and Cortex Radicis Moutan (*Dan Pi*) to cool the blood and stop bleeding.

If there is sticky, yellow phlegm which cannot be coughed up easily, add Pericarpium Trichosanthis Kirlowii (*Gua Lou Pi*) and Bulbus Fritillariae Thunbergii (*Zhe Bei Mu*) to clear and transform hot phlegm.

If there is cough with thick, yellow phlegm, add Fructus Trichosanthis Kirlowii (*Gua Lou*), Radix Scutellariae Baicalensis (*Huang Qin*), and Herba Houttuyniae Cordatae (*Yu Xing Cao*).

If there is a yellow tongue coating and thick, yellow phlegm, add Radix Scutellariae Baicalensis (*Huang Qin*) and Semen Benincasae Hispidae (*Dong Gua Ren*).

If there is sore throat, add Fructificatio Lasiosphaerae Seu Calvatiae (*Ma Bo*) and Fructus Arctii Lappae (*Niu Bang Zi*).

For severe sore throat as in acute tonsillitis, add Radix Scrophulariae Ningpoensis (*Xuan Shen*) and Fructus Arctii Lappae (*Niu Bang Zi*).

For wind heat affecting the eyes causing redness, itching, and pain, add Fructus Tribuli Terrestris (*Bai Ji Li*), Semen Cassiae Torae (*Jue Ming Zi*), and Spica Prunellae Vulgaris (*Xia Gu Cao*), or subtract Armeniaca and Platycodon and simply add Prunella and Cassia.

For heat entering the blood division, subtract Phragmites and Mint and add Tuber Ophiopogonis Japonicae (*Mai Dong*), raw Radix Rehmanniae (*Sheng Di*), Rhizoma Polygonati Odorati (*Yu Zhu*), and Cortex Radicis Moutan (*Dan Pi*).

For heat entering the constructive level with a dark red tongue, add Radix Scrophulariae Ningpoensis (*Xuan Shen*) and Cornu Rhinocerotis (*Xi Jiao*). Radix Arnebiae Seu Lithospermi (*Zi Cao*) or the combination of Radix Isatidis Seu Baphicacanthi (*Ban Lan Gen*) and Gypsum (*Shi Gao*) can be substituted for Rhinoceros Horn.

Comment: If fever is high and cough is severe, this formula may not be strong enough.

B. *Yin Qiao San* (Lonicera & Forsythia Powder)

Composition:

Fructus Forsythiae Suspensae (*Lian Qiao*), 9g
Flos Lonicerae Japonicae (*Yin Hua*), 9g
Radix Platycodi Grandiflori (*Ku Jie Geng*), 6g
Herba Menthae (*Bo He*), 6g
Folium Bambusae (*Zhu Ye*), 4g
raw Radix Glycyrrhizae (*Sheng Gan Cao*), 5g
Herba Seu Flos Schizonepetae Tenuifoliae (*Jing Jie Sui*), 5g
Semen Praeparatus Sojae (*Dan Dou Chi*), 5g
Fructus Arctii Lappae (*Niu Bang Zi*), 9g
Rhizoma Phragmitis Communis (*Lu Gen*), 9g

Functions: Acridly and cooly penetrates the exterior, clears heat and resolves toxins

Indications: Warm disease, initial stage. Common cold, flus, acute tonsillitis, mumps, measles, scarlatina, epidemic meningitis, encephalitis B, acute suppurative infections, and early stage sores.

Main signs & symptoms: Fever, no sweating or possible perspiration which does not flow easily, slight aversion to wind cold, headache, thirst, cough, sore throat, a red tongue tip and a thin, white or thin, yellow coating, and a floating, rapid pulse

Formula explanation:

The medicinals in this formula can be divided into three groups. First, Schizonepeta, Soja, and Mint emit perspiration, relieve the exterior, and resolve the muscles. Secondly, Lonicera, Forsythia, Folium Bambusae, and Phragmites clear heat and resolve toxins. Thirdly, Arctium, Platycodon, and Licorice stop cough, expel phlegm, and secure yin. In this formula, Lonicera and Forsythia are the sovereigns, which, being acrid and cool, penetrate evils, clear heat, and resolve toxins. Schizonepeta and Soja are the ministers. Although they are acrid and warm, they assist the sovereign medicinals in opening the skin and hair and dispelling evils. Platycodon and Arctium diffuse the lungs and disinhibit the throat. Licorice clears heat and resolves toxins. Folium Bambusae clears heat from the upper burner. Phragmites clears heat and engenders fluids. These are the assistant medicinals.

Additions & subtractions:

For high fever and sweating, subtract Schizonepeta and Soja and add Gypsum (*Shi Gao*) and Rhizoma Anemarrhenae (*Zhi Mu*).

For mumps, add Radix Isatidis Seu Baphicacanthi (*Ban Lan Gen*).

For heat and toxins, add both Radix Isatidis Seu Baphicacanthi (*Ban Lan Gen*) and Folium Isatidis (*Da Qing Ye*).

For early stage sores, add Herba Cum Radice Taraxaci Mongolici (*Pu Gong Ying*), Folium Isatidis (*Da Qing Ye*), and Herba Violae (*Zi Hua Di Ding*).

For a stifling sensation in the chest possibly accompanied by nausea and vomiting, add Herba Agastachis Seu Pogostemi (*Huo Xiang*) and Herba Eupatorii (*Pei Lan*).

If there is severe thirst, add Radix Trichosanthis Kirlowii (*Tian Hua Fen*).

If there is more serious sore throat, add Fructificatio Lasiosphaerae Seu Calvatiae (*Ma Bo*) and Radix Scrophulariae Ningpoensis (*Xuan Shen*).

Another option for the treatment of more serious sore throat is to add Radix Achyranthis Bidentatae (*Tu Niu Xi*), Radix Isatidis Seu Baphicacanthi (*Ban Lan Gen*), and Fructificatio Lasiosphaerae Seu Calvatiae (*Ma Bo*).

Yet another modification for sore throat consists of adding raw Radix Rehmanniae (*Sheng Di*) and Radix Scrophulariae Ningpoensis (*Xuan Shen*).

If there is more serious coughing, add Semen Pruni Armeniacae (*Xing Ren*) to disinhibit the lung qi. One can also add Folium Mori Albi (*Sang Ye*) along with the Armeniaca.

For cough with thick phlegm, add Semen Armeniacae (*Xing Ren*), Bulbus Fritillariae (*Bei Mu*), and Fructus Trichosanthis Kirlowii (*Gua Lou*).

If the disease has been harassing the lungs for 2-3 days and heat is now entering the interior, add raw Radix Rehmanniae (*Sheng Di*), and Tuber Ophiopogonis Japonicae (*Mai Dong*) to protect fluids and humors.

If this heat is not resolved and there is short urination, add Radix Scutellariae Baicalensis (*Huang Qin*), Rhizoma Anemarrhenae (*Zhi Mu*), and Fructus Gardeniae Jasminoidis (*Shan Zhi Zi*) plus the above two additions.

For nosebleed, subtract Schizonepeta and Soja and add Rhizoma Imperatae Cylindricae (*Bai Mao Gen*), carbonized Cacumen Biotae (*Ce Bai Tan*), and carbonized Fructus Gardeniae Jasminoidis (*Zhi Zi Tan*) to clear heat and cool the blood so as to stop bleeding.

If dampness is causing chest oppression and fullness and distention in the epigastrium, add Herba Agastachis Seu Pogostemi (*Huo Xiang*) and Tuber Curcumae (*Yu Jin*).

For early stage measles with rash not yet emitted, add Periostracum Cicadae (*Chan Tui*) and Herba Lemnae Seu Spirodelae (*Fu Ping*) or subtract Soja and add Radix Lithospermi Seu Arnebiae (*Zi Cao*) and Cicada Slough.

For measles rash not emitting fully, add Rhizoma Cimicifugae (*Sheng Ma*) and Radix Puerariae Lobatae (*Ge Gen*).

For early stage skin lesions, add Herba Cum Radice Taraxaci Mongolici (*Pu Gong Ying*) and Folium Isatidis (*Da Qing Ye*).

If there is a yellow tongue coating and diarrhea, add the ingredients of *Ge Gen Huang Lian Huang Qin Tang* (Pueraria, Scutellaria, and Coptis Decoction), *i.e.*, Radix Puerariae Lobatae (*Ge Gen*), Radix Scutellariae Baicalensis (*Huang Qin*), and Rhizoma Coptidis Chinensis (*Huang Lian*).

In order to dispel wind more effectively, add Radix Ledebouriellae Sesloidis (*Fang Feng*).

For frontal headache, add Radix Angelicae (*Bai Zhi*) and Flos Chrysanthemi Morifolii (*Ju Hua*).

For more severe heat, add Cortex Phellodendron (*Huang Bai*).

For qi vacuity, add Fructus Zizyphi Jujubae (*Da Zao*).

For stuffy nose, add Flos Magnoliae (*Xin Yi*) and Radix Puerariae Lobatae (*Ge Gen*).

Comment: This formula is similar in many ways to the preceding one. The key to distinguishing these is that *Yin Qiao San* is for exterior wind heat with fever and sore throat, while *Sang Ju Yin* is for exterior wind heat with less fever and toxins but more serious cough.

C. *Fu Zheng Jie Biao Ji* (Supporting the righteous, relieving the exterior formulas)

Representative formula: *Bai Du San* **(Vanquishing Toxins Powder)**

Composition:

Radix Bupleuri (*Chai Hu*)
Radix Peucedani (*Qian Hu*)
Rhizoma Ligustici Wallichii (*Chuan Xiong*)
Fructus Citri Seu Ponciri (*Zhi Ke*)
Radix Et Rhizoma Notopterygii (*Qiang Huo*)
Radix Angelicae Pubescentis (*Du Huo*)
Sclerotium Poriae Cocos (*Fu Ling*)
Radix Platycodi Grandiflori (*Jie Geng*), stir-fried
Radix Panacis Ginseng (*Ren Shen*)
Radix Glycyrrhizae (*Gan Cao*)

Method of administration: Grind equal amounts of the first 9 ingredients and half as much Licorice into a fine powder. Take 6g each time (cooked) with raw Rhizoma Zingiberis (*Sheng Jiang*) and Herba Menthae (*Bo He*). It may also be taken as a decoction without grinding the medicinals.

Functions: To emit perspiration and relieve the exterior, scatter wind and eliminate dampness while simultaneously boosting the qi

Indications: Common cold, wind, cold, damp evils. Upper respiratory tract infections, flus, emphysema, malaria, early stage dysentery, early stage measles, acute cellulitis, and sores

Main signs & symptoms: Abhorrence of cold, high fever, stiffness and pain of the head and neck, aching and pain of the body and limbs, no sweating, stuffed nose, a hoarse voice, cough with phlegm, chest and diaphragm glomus and fullness, a slimy, white tongue coating, and a floating, soggy or floating, relaxed/retarded pulse. If the case is more serious, the pulse may be forceless.

Contraindications:

1. Because many of the medicinals in this formula are warm, windy, and drying, this formula should only be used for the treatment of exterior pattern wind, cold, and dampness. It is contraindicated in cases where there is heat.

Formula explanation:

Notopterygium and *Du Huo* are the sovereigns. They are acrid, warm, emitting, and scattering. They open and treat the entire body, above and below, for wind, cold, damp evils. Ligusticum moves the blood and eliminates wind. Bupleurum, acrid and scattering, relieves the muscles. These are the minister medicinals. They assist Notopterygium and *Du Huo* in eliminating external evils and stopping aching and pain. Citrus downbears the qi. Platycodon opens the lungs. Peucedanum eliminates phlegm. Poria percolates dampness. These are the assistant medicinals. They disinhibit the lung qi, eliminate phlegm dampness, and stop coughing. Licorice regulates and harmonizes these medicinals. It simultaneously boosts the qi and harmonizes the stomach. Ginger and Mint emit and scatter wind cold. These two are the messenger ingredients. All these are combined with a small amount of Ginseng to supplement the qi. When the righteous qi is sufficient, evils are blown and exited outside. With one sweat, wind, cold, and dampness are all dispelled. Ginseng is also an assistant medicinal.

Additions & subtractions:

For malarial diseases, increase the amount of Bupleurum and add Radix Scutellariae Baicalensis (*Huang Qin*) and Semen Arecae Catechu (*Bing Lang*).

During the initial stage of an ulcerous swelling, add Herba Seu Flos Schizonepetae Tenuifoliae (*Jing Jie*) and Radix Ledebouriellae Sesloidis (*Fang Feng*). This results in *Jing Fang Bai Du San* (Schizonepeta & Ledebouriella Vanquishing Toxins Powder).

For early stage sores which are red, swollen, and painful and accompanied by other signs and symptoms of exterior patterns, add Flos Lonicerae Japonicae (*Yin Hua*) and Fructus Forsythiae Suspensae (*Lian Qiao*). This results in *Yin Qiao Bai Du San* (Lonicera & Forsythia Vanquishing Toxins Powder). If there is no obvious vacuity, subtract Ginseng.

For the initial stage of dysentery, subtract Ginseng and add Radix Saussureae Seu Vladimiriae (*Mu Xiang*) and Rhizoma Coptidis Chinensis (*Huang Lian*).

For chattering mouth dysentery with toxic qi penetrating the heart and hot vomiting, subtract Bupleurum and add old, stored rice (*Chen Cang Mi*). This results in *Cang Lin San* (Granary Powder).

For external invasion, wind cold with internal phlegm rheum, aversion to cold, fever, headache, stuffed nose, cough with copious phlegm, chest and diaphragm fullness and oppression, a white tongue coating, and a slippery pulse, subtract Ligusticum, *Du Huo*, and Notopterygium and add Rhizoma Pinelliae Ternatae (*Ban Xia*), Folium Perillae Frutescentis (*Su Ye*), Radix Puerariae Lobatae (*Ge Gen*), Pericarpium

19

Citri Reticulatae (*Chen Pi*), Radix Saussurea Seu Vladimiriae (*Mu Xiang*), raw Rhizoma Zingiberis (*Sheng Jiang*), and Fructus Zizyphi Jujubae (*Da Zao*). This results in *Shen Su Yin* (Ginseng & Perilla Drink).

If there is no cough, subtract Platycodon and Peucedanum and add Ramulus Mori Albi (*Sang Zhi*) and Ramus Lonicerae Japonicae (*Ren Dong Teng*).

If there is severe cough, subtract Notopterygium, *Du Huo*, and Ligusticum and add Rhizoma Pinelliae Ternatae (*Ban Xia*), Radix Asteris Tartarici (*Zi Wan*), and Radix Stemonae (*Bai Bu*).

2

Xie Xia Ji
Draining & Precipitating Formulas

Draining and precipitating formulas are used to treat interior repletion patterns when turbid qi is unable to descend due to internal accumulation of evil qi. In this case, typically there will be epigastric and/or lower abdominal distention, loss of appetite, constipation, and abdominal pain aggravated by pressure. Precipitating medicinals open and conduct the large intestine and eliminate accumulations and stagnation from the stomach and intestines. These can consist of replete heat, water rheum, or accumulation of cold. Thus there are three subcategories of draining and precipitating formulas which purge replete evils through the bowels. These are 1) cold precipitating formulas, 2) warm precipitating formulas, and 3) water-dispelling precipitating formulas. Cold precipitating formulas use cold natured medicinals to drain and precipitate replete heat. Warm precipitating formulas use warm medicinals combined with draining and precipitating medicinals. They are for the treatment of cold binding interior repletion patterns causing constipation and abdominal fullness and distention. Water-dispelling precipitating formulas use harsh cathartics to drain via the bowels and urination water rheum gathering and accumulating in the interior causing repletion patterns. In addition, there is also the subcategory of moistening precipitating formulas for the treatment of fluid dryness constipation.

Cautions & Contraindications When Using Draining & Precipitating Medicinals

1. Do not drain and precipitate when exterior patterns have not yet been relieved nor when interior symptoms are not serious.
2. Do not drain and precipitate pregnant women nor postpartum except with great care.
3. Do not drain during prolonged illness with bodily weakness nor in the elderly except with great care.
4. When the evil is eliminated, draining and precipitation must stop. Do not overdose.

2.1 *Han Xia Ji* (Cold precipitating formulas)

Representative formula: *Da Cheng Qi Tang* (Great Order the Qi Decoction)

Composition:

Radix Et Rhizoma Rhei (*Da Huang*), 12g
Cortex Magnoliae Officinalis (*Hou Po*), 15g, remove skin, mix-fried
Fructus Immaturus Citri Seu Ponciri (*Zhi Shi*), 12g
Mirabilitum (*Mang Xiao*), 9g

Method of preparation: Decoct the Magnolia and Immature Citrus first. Only add the Rhubarb during the last several minutes of cooking. Prolonged cooking reduces Rhubarb's effectiveness as a purgative. Then Mirabilitum is stirred in and dissolved after the decoction has been strained.

Functions: Sternly (or harshly) precipitates heat binding

Indications: 1) *Yang ming* bowel repletion patterns, 2) heat binding circumfluence, and 3) interior heat repletion patterns of heat inversion.

Acute pneumonia, typhoid, flus, measles, meningitis, hypertension, tetanus, beriberi, habitual constipation, appendicitis, intestinal obstruction, acute abdominal pain, neurosis, food poisoning, obesity, dysentery, hemorrhoids

Main signs & symptoms: 1) Constipation, high fever, epigastric glomus and fullness, pain in the abdomen which dislikes pressure, if severe, tidal fever, delirious speech, and profuse sweating from the hands and feet, a dry, yellow, prickly tongue coating which may even be charred black and dry, and a deep, replete pulse; 2) precipitation of clear, green colored water, abdominal pain, a hard, lumpy feeling on pressure, a dry mouth and tongue, and a slippery, replete pulse; and 3) epileptic or convulsive diseases or mania.

Contraindications:

1. If inappropriately prescribed, this formula may cause vomiting and severe diarrhea.
2. It is generally prohibited during pregnancy.

Formula explanation:

In this formula, Rhubarb is the sovereign medicinal. It drains heat and opens the bowels, sweeps and washes the stomach and intestines. Mirabilitum assists Rhubarb drain heat and open the bowels. It is also able to soften the hard and moisten dryness. It is the minister medicinal. These two medicinals together sternly precipitate heat binding and their strength is very great. If there are accumulations and stagnation obstructing within, the bowel qi is not free flowing. Therefore, Citrus Immaturus and Magnolia move the qi and scatter nodulation, disperse glomus and eliminate fullness. Hence they assist Rhubarb and Mirabilitum sweep away accumulation and stagnation and are the assistant medicinals.

Additions & subtractions:

If *yang ming* bowel repletion is relatively mild or there is mild damage of fluids and humors, subtract Mirabilitum. This results in *Xiao Cheng Qi Tang* (Minor Order the Qi Decoction).

If there is severe fluid dryness of the intestines as manifest by constipation, subtract Magnolia and Citrus Immaturus and add Radix Scrophulariae Ningpoensis (*Yuan Shen*), raw Radix Rehmanniae (*Sheng Di*), and Tuber Ophiopogonis Japonicae (*Mai Dong*). This results in *Zeng Ye Cheng Qi Tang* (Increase Fluids & Order the Qi Decoction).

If there is no glomus or abdominal fullness but mild constipation with irritability and a slippery, rapid pulse, subtract Citrus Immaturus and Magnolia and add mix-fried Radix Glycyrrhizae (*Zhi Gan Cao*). This results in *Tiao Wei Cheng Qi Tang* (Regulate the Stomach Order the Qi Decoction).

If there is more serious abdominal pain, distention, constipation, and vomiting, add Semen Pruni Persicae (*Tao Ren*), Radix Rubrus Paeoniae Lactiflorae (*Chi Shao*), and stir-fried Semen Raphani Sativi (*Chao Lai Fu Zi*). This results in *Fu Fang Da Cheng Qi Tang* (Compound Great Order the Qi Decoction).

For high fever, extreme thirst, and a rapid, forceful pulse, add Rhizoma Anemarrhenae (*Zhi Mu*) and Gypsum (*Shi Gao*).

For severe abdominal distention, fullness, and pain, add Semen Raphani Sativi (*Lai Fu Zi*), Semen Pruni Persicae (*Tao Ren*), and Radix Rubrus Paeoniae Lactiflorae (*Chi Shao*).

For signs of blood stasis, add Radix Rubrus Paeoniae Lactiflorae (*Chi Shao*) and Semen Pruni Persicae (*Tao Ren*).

For severe bloating, add Radix Saussureae Seu Vladimiriae (*Mu Xiang*) and Semen Arecae Catechu (*Bing Lang*).

For delirium, add Ramulus Uncariae Cum Uncis (*Gou Teng*) and Sclerotium Pararadicis Poriae Cocos (*Fu Shen*).

If there is concomitant liver depression, qi stagnation, add Radix Bupleuri (*Chai Hu*), Radix Scutellariae Baicalensis (*Huang Qin*), and Radix Paeoniae Lactiflorae (*Shao Yao*).

For peritonitis, subtract Mirabilitum and add Rhizoma Pinelliae Ternatae (*Ban Xia*) and raw Rhizoma Zingiberis (*Sheng Jiang*).

For exterior cold patterns with interior heat accompanied by constipation and bloating, subtract Mirabilitum and add Ramulus Cinnamomi (*Gui Zhi*), raw Rhizoma Zingiberis (*Sheng Jiang*), Fructus Zizyphi Jujubae (*Da Zao*), and Radix Glycyrrhizae (*Gan Cao*). This results in *Hou Po Qi Wu Tang* (Magnolia Seven Materials Decoction).

For women's lower abdominal blood stasis with heat binding, add Flos Carthami Tinctorii (*Hong Hua*), Radix Angelicae Sinensis (*Dang Gui*), and Radix Glycyrrhizae (*Gan Cao*). This results in *Da Huang Hou Po Tang* (Rhubarb & Magnolia Decoction).

If there is severe qi and blood vacuity, add Radix Panacis Ginseng (*Ren Shen*) and Radix Angelicae Sinensis (*Dang Gui*). This results in *Huang Long Tang* (Yellow Dragon Decoction).

2.2 *Wen Xia Ji* (Warm precipitating formulas)

Representative formula: *Da Huang Fu Zi Tang* (Rhubarb & Aconite Decoction)

Composition:

Radix Et Rhizoma Rhei (*Da Huang*), 9g
Radix Praeparatus Aconiti Carmichaeli (*Fu Zi*), 9g, blast-fried
Herba Cum Radice Asari (*Xi Xin*), 3g

Functions: Warms yang and scatters cold, drains binding and moves stagnation

Indications: Cold accumulation interior repletion. Stomach and intestinal spasms, pyelonephritis, kidney stones, gallstones, pancreatitis, intestinal colic, hernia pain, sciatica, intercostal neuralgia, migraines, chronic colitis, and chronic pelvic inflammation.

Main signs & symptoms: Abdominal pain and constipation, lateral costal and one-sided hypochondrial pain, fever, counterflow inversion of the hands and feet (*i.e.*, chilled hands and feet), a white, slimy tongue coating, and a tight, wiry pulse

Formula explanation:

In this formula, Aconite is acrid and warm. It warms yang in order to dispel cold. It is assisted by Asarum which eliminates cold and scatters nodulation. Rhubarb sweeps away and washes clear the stomach and intestines, drains and eliminates accumulations and stagnation. Thus, with accumulated cold scattered and the stools moving, interior repletion is eliminated, the bowel qi flows freely, and hence abdominal pain, fever, and counterflow of the limbs are entirely leveled.

Additions & subtractions:

For severe abdominal pain, add Ramulus Cinnamomi (*Gui Zhi*) and Radix Albus Paeoniae Lactiflorae (*Bai Shao*).

For severe distention and a thick, slimy tongue coating, add Fructus Immaturus Citri Seu Ponciri (*Zhi Shi*) and Massa Medica Fermentata (*Shen Qu*).

For severe abdominal fullness, add Cortex Magnoliae Officinalis (*Hou Po*) and Radix Saussureae Seu Vladimiriae (*Mu Xiang*).

If there is only mild accumulation or in patients with bodily weakness and vacuity, use processed Radix Et Rhizoma Rhei (*Zhi Da Huang*).

For cold *shan* with severe pain in the low back and inguinal regions, add Cortex Cinnamomi (*Rou Gui*) and Fructus Foeniculi Vulgaris (*Xiao Hui Xiang*).

For spleen vacuity with cold accumulation and constipation, abdominal pain, chilled extremities, and a deep, wiry pulse, subtract Asarum and add Radix Panacis Ginseng (*Ren Shen*), mix-fried Radix Glycyrrhizae (*Zhi Gan Cao*), and dry Rhizoma Zingiberis (*Gan Jiang*). This results in *Wen Pi Tang* (Warm the Spleen Decoction).

For bodily weakness, add Radix Codonopsis Pilosulae (*Dang Shen*) and Radix Angelicae Sinensis (*Dang Gui*) to boost the qi and nourish the blood.

Comment: Patients requiring this kind of formula are often complicated and typically manifest a combination of repletion and vacuity patterns.

2.3 *Zhui Shui Ji* (Water-expelling formulas)

Representative formula: *Shi Zao Tang* (Ten Dates Decoction)

Composition:

Radix Euphorbiae Kansui (*Gan Sui*)
Radix Euphorbiae Seu Knoxiae (*Da Ji*)
Flos Daphnis Genkwae (*Yuan Hua*)

Method of preparation & administration: Grind equal amounts of the above medicinals into a fine powder and take 0.5-1g in the early morning on an empty stomach. Follow this with a warm decoction made from 10 pieces of Fructus Zizyphi Jujubae (*Da Zao*), thus the name of this formula. Except for Red Dates, these ingredients will lose their effectiveness if cooked.

One half to one hour after taking, there will be upper abdominal discomfort and mild dizziness and nausea followed by loose stools. If there is no bowel movement after 1 hour, take a second dose. If the bowel movements are too frequent, eat cold rice soup.

Functions: Attacks and drives out water rheum

Indications: 1) Suspended rheum and 2) replete water. Tuberculous exudative pleurisy, rheumatic pleurisy, ascites due to cirrhosis, schistosomiasis, nephritis, or uremia from systemic lupus erythematosus.

Main signs & symptoms: 1) Cough causing pain in the chest and lateral costal regions, hard glomus beneath the heart, dry heaves and shortness of breath, headache, vertigo, possible chest pain extending to the upper back with the pain making breathing difficult, a white

28

tongue coating, and a deep, wiry pulse; 2) swelling of the entire body which is worse in the lower extremities, abdominal distention, wheezing, and fullness, and inhibition of urination and defecation.

Contraindications:

1. Do not use this formula in patients with bodily weakness and vacuity.
2. Do not use during pregnancy.
3. If diarrhea ensues, take cold rice porridge.

Formula explanation:

In this formula, Euphorbia Kansui moves the channels and tunnels away water dampness. Euphorbia Seu Knoxia discharges water dampness from the viscera and bowels. Daphnes disperses hidden rheum phlegm conglomerations from the chest and lateral costal regions. When these three medicinals are used together, they are very harsh and attacking. Their ability to drive out water rheum, eliminate accumulations and gatherings, disperse swelling and fullness is extreme. With the channels tunneled (open), accumulated water in the viscera and bowels, chest and lateral costal regions is expelled. Because these three medicinals used together easily damage the righteous qi, Red Dates, which are sweet, are taken to boost the qi and protect the stomach. They are able to moderate and harmonize the harsh, toxic nature of these other medicinals so that there can be precipitation without damaging the righteous.

Comment: This is a very strong formula which should only be used when absolutely necessary. In cases suffering from concomitant vacuity weakness, this formula can be alternated with a supplementing formula to support the righteous.

2.4 *Ru Xia Ji* (Moistening & precipitating formulas)

Representative formula: *Ma Zi Ren Wan* (Cannabis Seed Pills)

Composition:

Semen Cannabis Sativae (*Huo Ma Ren*), 500g
Radix Paeoniae Lactiflorae (*Shao Yao*), 250g
Fructus Immaturus Citri Seu Ponciri (*Zhi Shi*), 250g, mix-fried
Radix Et Rhizoma Rhei (*Da Huang*), 500g, remove the skin
Cortex Magnoliae Officinalis (*Hou Po*), 250g, mix-fried, remove the skin
Semen Pruni Armeniacae (*Xing Ren*), 250g, remove the tip and skin

Method of administration: Grind the above 6 medicinals into fine powder and mix with honey to form pills. Take 9g each time, 1-2 times per day with warm water. This formula can also be taken as a decoction, in which case one should reduce the dosages proportionately.

Functions: Moistens the intestines and discharges heat, moves the qi and opens the bowels

Indications: Stomach and intestines dry heat, fluids and humors insufficient. Constipation in those who are either aged or bodily weak and vacuous, postpartum or post-surgical constipation, habitual constipation, chronic colitis, or hemorrhoids.

Main signs & symptoms: Stools dry and knotted, urination short and frequent, a dry, yellow tongue coating, and a floating, rapid pulse

Contraindications:

1. Do not use during pregnancy.

Cannabis Seeds are the sovereign medicinal in this formula. They moisten the intestines and open the bowels. Rhubarb opens the bowels and discharges heat. Armeniaca downbears the qi and moistens the intestines. White Peony nourishes yin and harmonizes the interior. These are the minister medicinals. Citrus Immaturus and Magnolia precipitate the qi and crack binding. Additionally, they have a strong power to downbear, discharge, and open the bowels. Honey is able to moisten dryness and lubricate the intestines. These are the assistant medicinals.

Additions & subtractions:

For hemorrhoids due to blood stasis, add Semen Pruni Persicae (*Tao Ren*) and Radix Angelicae Sinensis (*Dang Gui*).

For bleeding hemorrhoids, add Flos Immaturus Sophorae Japonicae (*Huai Hua*) and Radix Sanguisorbae (*Di Yu*).

If damage to fluids and humors is severe, add Semen Biotae Orientalis (*Bai Zi Ren*) and Semen Trichosanthis Kirlowii (*Gua Lou Ren*).

If heat accumulation is severe with a yellow tongue coating and rapid pulse, increase the amount of Rhubarb and add Mirabilitum (*Mang Xiao*).

For severe vacuity weakness, subtract Rhubarb and add a small amount of Folium Sennae (*Fan Xie Ye*).

For central qi vacuity, take with *Bu Zhong Yi Qi Tang* (Supplement the Center, Boost the Qi Decoction).

For intestinal obstruction due to roundworms, add Fructus Pruni Mume (*Wu Mei*), Semen Arecae Catechu (*Bing Lang*), and Pericarpium Citri Reticulatae (*Chen Pi*).

Comment: Once constipation has been relieved, the use of these pills should be stopped since it is not good to take Rhubarb habitually.

3

He Jie Ji
Harmonizing & Resolving Formulas

Harmonizing and resolving (or relieving) formulas are those which regulate and harmonize. Typically, they support the righteous while simultaneously attacking evil. There are three subcategories of harmonizing and resolving formulas: 1) formulas which harmonize and resolve the *shao yang*, 2) formulas which regulate and harmonize the liver and spleen, and 3) formulas which regulate and harmonize the stomach and intestines. The first subcategory of harmonizing formulas is used in order to relieve and eliminate *shao yang* half exterior/half interior evils. The second subcategory is used when the functions of the liver and spleen have lost their regularity. The third subcategory is used when cold and heat above and below are mutually binding.

3.1 *He Jie Shao Yang Ji* (Formulas which harmonize & resolve the *shao yang*)

Representative formula: *Xiao Chai Hu Tang* (Minor Bupleurum Decoction)

Composition:

Radix Bupleuri (*Chai Hu*), 12g
Radix Scutellariae Baicalensis (*Huang Qin*), 9g
Radix Panacis Ginseng (*Ren Shen*), 6g
Rhizoma Pinelliae Ternatae (*Ban Xia*), 9g

Radix Glycyrrhizae (*Gan Cao*), 5g, mix-fried
raw Rhizoma Zingiberis (*Sheng Jiang*), 9g
Fructus Zizyphi Jujubae (*Da Zao*), 4 pieces

Functions: Harmonizes and resolves the *shao yang*

Indications: 1) Cold damage *shao yang* patterns and 2) women's damage by cold. Common cold with lingering fever after several days, acute and chronic bronchitis, pleuritis, pneumonia, pulmonary tuberculosis, sinusitis, malaria, hepatitis, both acute viral and chronic, cholecystitis, gallstones, jaundice, gastritis, gastric ulcer, stomachache, lymphadenitis, tonsillitis, otitis media, mumps, mastitis, intercostal neuralgia, torticollis, pyelonephritis, puerperal fever, severe chills and fever due to uterine disease, stuttering, epilepsy, impotence in young men, neurosis, alopecia, and mental instability in children.

Main signs & symptoms: Alternating fever and chills, chest and lateral costal region bitterness (*i.e.*, pain) and fullness, diminished intake of food and drink, heart vexation, a desire to vomit, acid eructations, possible jaundice, a bitter (taste) in the mouth, a dry throat, vertigo, a thin, white tongue coating, and a wiry pulse.

Contraindications:

1. Do not use in patients with repletion above and vacuity below.
2. Do not use in case of liver fire and bleeding gums.
3. Use cautiously with patients with hyperactivity of liver yang, hypertension, of vomiting of blood due to yin vacuity.
4. Use cautiously with patients with headache and dizziness.

Formula explanation:

Within this formula, Bupleurum is the particular medicinal which enters the *shao yang*. It gently clears, upbears, and scatters. It also courses evils and penetrates the exterior. Thus it is the sovereign medicinal in this formula. Scutellaria is bitter and cold. It clears *shao yang* ministerial fire. It is the minister medicinal. Combined with Bupleurum, one scatters and the other clears, thus resolving *shao yang* evils. Pinellia harmonizes the stomach and downbears counterflow, scatters nodulation and disperses glomus. It is the assistant medicinal. It assists both the sovereign and minister medicinals attack evils. Ginseng and Licorice are also assistants, while Ginger and Red Dates are the messengers. They boost stomach qi, engender fluids and humors, harmonize the constructive and defensive, and support the righteous in order to help dispel evils. They also replenish the interior so that evils cannot enter it.

Additions & subtractions:

If there is pronounced thirst, subtract Pinellia and add Radix Trichosanthis Kirlowii (*Tian Hua Fen*).

If there is no vomiting, subtract Pinellia and Ginseng and add Fructus Trichosanthis Kirlowii (*Gua Lou*).

If there is abdominal pain, subtract Scutellaria and add Radix Albus Paeoniae Lactiflorae (*Bai Shao*).

Also for abdominal pain, add Fructus Amomi (*Sha Ren*) and Radix Saussureae Seu Vladimiriae (*Mu Xiang*).

Again for abdominal distention and pain, add Rhizoma Corydalis Yanhusuo (*Yan Hu*), Rhizoma Cyperi Rotundi (*Xiang Fu*), and Fructus Immaturus Citri Seu Ponciri (*Zhi Shi*).

For distention and pain of the lower abdomen, subtract Ginseng and Licorice and add Rhizoma Cyperi Rotundi (*Xiang Fu*) and Fructus Citri Seu Ponciri (*Zhi Ke*).

For scanty, reddish yellow, astringent, and painful urination, add Herba Desmodii (*Jin Qian Cao*) and Herba Oldenlandiae (*Bai Hua She She Cao*).

For fever, aversion to wind, headache, chest fullness and oppression, constipation, loss of appetite, reddish yellow urine, irritability, thirst, a yellow tongue coating, and a tight pulse, add Semen Cannabis Sativae (*Huo Ma Ren*) and Fructus Immaturus Citri Seu Ponciri (*Zhi Shi*).

For fever, cough with yellow phlegm, and pain in the chest, add Radix Platycodi Grandiflori (*Jie Geng*), Fructus Trichosanthis Kirlowii (*Gua Lou*), and Bulbus Fritillariae Cirrhosae (*Chuan Bei Mu*).

For malarial diseases, add Herba Artemisiae Apiaceae (*Qing Hao*) and Radix Dichroae Febrifugae (*Chang Shan*).

Also for malarial diseases, add Radix Dichroae Febrifugae (*Chang Shan*) and Fructus Amomi Tsaokuo (*Cao Guo*).

For malarial diseases with a heavy sensation in the limbs, loss of appetite, and a soggy pulse, subtract Ginger and Red Dates and add Rhizoma Atractylodis (*Cang Zhu*) and Cortex Magnoliae Officinalis (*Hou Po*). This results in *Chai Ping Tang* (Bupleurum Levelling Decoction).

For vertigo, add Flos Chrysanthemi Morifolii (*Ju Hua*), Ramulus Uncariae Seu Uncis (*Gou Teng*), and Semen Cassiae Torae (*Jue Ming Zi*).

For coughs which are worse at midnight, alternating fever and chills, and a bitter taste in the mouth, add dry Rhizoma Zingiberis (*Gan Jiang*), Herba Cum Radice Asari (*Xi Xin*), and Fructus Schizandrae Chinensis (*Wu Wei Zi*).

For urinary tract infections with chills, fever, and urgent, frequent urination, take with *Liu Wei Di Huang Wan* (Six Flavored Rehmannia Pills).

For concomitant yin vacuity, add Carapax Amydae (*Bie Jia*) and Herba Artemisiae Apiaceae (*Qing Hao*).

For chest oppression and epigastric fullness, add Rhizoma Cyperi Rotundi (*Xiang Fu*) and Fructus Immaturus Citri Seu Ponciri (*Zhi Shi*).

For concomitant kidney yang vacuity with cockcrow diarrhea, lower abdominal bloating, and thirst, add Sclerotium Poriae Cocos (*Fu Ling*), Rhizoma Alismatis (*Ze Xie*), Radix Dioscoreae Oppositae (*Shan Yao*), and Semen Cuscutae (*Tu Si Zi*).

For lung qi and exterior vacuity, add Fructus Schizandrae Chinensis (*Wu Wei Zi*) and Radix Astragali Membranacei (*Huang Qi*).

For recurrent lung heat diseases, add Rhizoma Coptidis Chinensis (*Huang Lian*) and Semen Trichosanthis Kirlowii (*Gua Lou Ren*). This results in *Chai Xian Tang* (Bupleurum Fall Decoction).

For cough with sticky, hard to expectorate phlegm, add Semen Trichosanthis Kirlowii (*Gua Lou Ren*), Radix Platycodi Grandiflori (*Jie Geng*), and Fructus Immaturus Citri Seu Ponciri (*Zhi Shi*).

For dry cough, add Tuber Ophiopogonis Japonicae (*Mai Dong*) and Caulis In Taeniis Bambusae (*Zhu Ru*).

For sinusitis with a yellow nasal discharge due to gallbladder heat invading the brain, add Fructus Xanthii (*Cang Er Zi*).

For muscle tension and chronic intestinal disorders with chilled extremities, add Ramulus Cinnamomi (*Gui Zhi*) and Radix Albus

37

Paeoniae Lactiflorae (*Bai Shao*). This results in *Chai Hu Gui Zhi Tang* (Bupleurum & Cinnamon Decoction).

For pleurisy and atony diseases involving the lungs, add Radix Gentianae Macrophyllae (*Qin Jiao*), Cortex Radicis Lycii (*Di Gu Pi*), Radix Asteris Tartarici (*Zi Wan*), Carapax Amydae (*Bie Jia*), Radix Angelicae Sinensis (*Dang Gui*), and Fructus Pruni Mume (*Wu Mei*). This results in *Qin Jiao Fu Lei Tang* (Gentiana Macrophylla Support Marked Emaciation Decoction).

If there is constipation, add Mirabilitum (*Mang Xiao*). This results in *Chai Hu Jia Mang Xiao Tang* (Bupleurum & Mirabilitum Decoction).

If there is alternating fever and chills, headache in the lateral sides of the forehead, vertigo, fullness and pain in the chest and lateral costal regions, a white tongue coating, and a wiry, slippery pulse on the right and a wiry, floating, large pulse on the left, subtract Ginseng and Red Dates and add Fructus Citri Seu Ponciri (*Zhi Ke*), Radix Platycodi Grandiflori (*Jie Geng*), and Pericarpium Citri Reticulatae (*Chen Pi*). This results in *Chai Hu Zhi Jie Tang* (Bupleurum, Citrus, & Platycodon Decoction).

If a female patient catches a cold before or with each period accompanied by alternating fever and chills, lack of appetite, and a wiry pulse, add the ingredients of *Si Wu Tang* (Four Materials Decoction).

For constipation or diarrhea which burns the anus, abdominal glomus and fullness which feels hard to the touch, nausea, continuous vomiting, a bitter taste in the mouth, despondency and slight irritability, a yellow tongue coating, and a wiry, forceful pulse, subtract Ginseng and add Radix Et Rhizoma Rhei (*Da Huang*), Radix Albus Paeoniae Lactiflorae (*Bai Shao*), and Fructus Immaturus Citri Seu Ponciri (*Zhi Shi*). This results in *Da Chai Hu Tang* (Major Bupleurum Decoction).

If there is severe vomiting and constipation, to *Da Chai Hu Tang* add Rhizoma Coptidis Chinensis (*Huang Lian*) and Fructus Evodiae Rutecarpae (*Wu Zhu Yu*).

If there is severe pain and constipation, to *Da Chai Hu Tang* add Radix Angelicae Sinensis (*Dang Gui*) and Rhizoma Corydalis Yanhusuo (*Yan Hu*) or Radix Rubrus Paeoniae Lactiflorae (*Chi Shao*) and Semen Pruni Persicae (*Tao Ren*).

For evil heat entering the blood chamber, add Folium Perillae Frutescentis (*Zi Su Ye*).

For menstrual irregularity and premenstrual tension, add Rhizoma Cyperi Rotundi (*Xiang Fu*) and Radix Albus Paeoniae Lactiflorae (*Bai Shao*).

For premenstrual breast distention, add Fructus Meliae Toosendan (*Chuan Lian Zi*) and Spica Prunellae Vulgaris (*Xia Gu Cao*).

For vexatious heat before the period, reduce the dosages of Pinellia and Ginseng and add Cortex Radicis Moutan (*Dan Pi*), Fructus Gardeniae Jasminoidis (*Shan Zhi Zi*), and raw Radix Rehmanniae (*Sheng Di*).

For premenstrual edema, add Sclerotium Poriae Cocos (*Fu Ling*) and Rhizoma Alismatis (*Ze Xie*).

For premenstrual palpitations and insomnia, add Radix Polygalae Tenuifoliae (*Yuan Zhi*), Semen Zizyphi Spinosae (*Suan Zao Ren*), and Radix Angelicae Sinensis (*Dang Gui*).

For premenstrual mental dullness and headache, add Flos Chrysanthemi Morifolii (*Ju Hua*) and Rhizoma Ligustici Wallichii (*Chuan Xiong*).

For clots in the menstruate, add Radix Salviae Miltiorrhizae (*Dan Shen*) and Caulis Millettiae Seu Spatholobi (*Ji Xue Teng*).

For infertility, add Fluoritum (*Zi Shi Ying*) and Fructus Ligustri Lucidi (*Nu Zhen Zi*).

Comment: Because many chronic diseases are a combination of repletion and vacuity, this formula has a very wide range of applicability. It is one of the most famous and most often used in all of Chinese medicine. It can be widely modified and is also commonly used for prevention and long-term health protection.

3.2 *Tiao He Gan Pi Ji* (Regulating & harmonizing the liver & spleen formulas)

Representative formulas:

A. *Si Ni San* (Four Counterflows Powder)

Composition:

Radix Glycyrrhizae (*Gan Cao*), 6g, mix-fried
Fructus Immaturus Citri Seu Ponciri (*Zhi Shi*), 9g, broken up, soaked
    in water, and mix-fried dry
Radix Bupleuri (*Chai Hu*), 9g
Radix Paeoniae Lactiflorae (*Shao Yao*), 12g

Functions: Penetrates the exterior and resolves depression, courses the liver and rectifies the spleen

Indications: *Shao yin* disease, four counterflows patterns (*i.e.*, cold extremities due to the liver failing to course and discharge heat). Gastritis, peptic ulcer, cholecystitis, gallstones, hepatitis, intercostal neuralgia, biliary ascariasis, hernia, acute appendicitis, pancreatitis, intestinal obstruction, allergic colitis, neurotic diarrhea, pleurisy, rhinitis, tubercular peritonitis, neurosis, epilepsy, mastitis, and fibrocystic breasts

Main signs & symptoms: Cold extremities, irritability, abdominal pain and distention, possible fever, possible palpitations, possible inhibited urination, possible severe diarrhea, tenesmus, menstrual irregularity in women, a red tongue with a yellow coating, and a wiry, rapid pulse

Contraindications:

1. Do not use in cold collapse, vacuity desertion, or shock.
2. Do not use to treat liver yin vacuity (without modification).
3. Do not use to treat vacuity cold of central warmer (without modification).
4. Reduce the dosage of Licorice in the presence of marked abdominal distention.

Formula explanation:

Within this formula, mix-fried Licorice, sweet and warm, boosts the qi so as to fortify the spleen. It also harmonizes the other medicinals in this formula. Bupleurum penetrates the exterior and upbears yang so as to soothe depression. At the same time, because it is acrid and cool, it clears internal heat by out-thrusting it. Citrus Immaturus precipitates the qi and cracks nodulation, and, when it is combined with Bupleurum, the upbearing and downbearing of the qi is regulated, thus also regulating the spleen and stomach. Peony boosts yin and nourishes the blood, harmonizes the liver and stops pain. Combined with Bupleurum, the two course the liver and rectify the spleen. By combining all four ingredients, evils are expelled and depression resolved, qi and blood are regulated and smoothed, clear yang begets the spirit, and the four counterflows are automatically cured.

Additions & subtractions:

For cough, add Fructus Schizandrae Chinensis (*Wu Wei Zi*) and dry Rhizoma Zingiberis (*Gan Jiang*) to warm the lungs and scatter cold.

For palpitations, add Ramulus Cinnamomi (*Gui Zhi*) to warm yang and disinhibit water.

For inhibited urination, add Sclerotium Poriae Cocos (*Fu Ling*) to blandly percolate and fortify the spleen in order to disinhibit water.

For vomiting, add *Zuo Jin Wan* (Left Gold Pills), *i.e.*, Rhizoma Coptidis Chinensis (*Huang Lian*) and Fructus Evodiae Rutecarpae (*Wu Zhu Yu*).

For upper abdominal pain with acid regurgitation, also add *Zuo Jin Wan* (Left Metal Pills).

For cold abdominal pain, add Radix Praeparatus Aconiti Carmichaeli (*Fu Zi*) to warm the center and scatter cold and thus stop pain.

For severe abdominal pain, add Rhizoma Cyperi Rotundi (*Xiang Fu*), Pericarpium Viridis Citri Reticulatae (*Qing Pi*), and Rhizoma Ligustici Wallichii (*Chuan Xiong*). This results in *Chai Hu Xiang Fu Tang* (Bupleurum & Cyperus Decoction).

For concomitant blood vacuity, add Radix Angelicae Sinensis (*Dang Gui*).

For blood vacuity with lateral costal pain and menstrual irregularity, subtract Citrus Immaturus and add Rhizoma Atractylodis Macrocephalae (*Bai Zhu*), Sclerotium Poriae Cocos (*Fu Ling*), and Radix Angelicae Sinensis (*Dang Gui*).

For severe lateral costal pain, add Tuber Curcumae (*Yu Jin*), Rhizoma Cyperi Rotundi (*Xiang Fu*), and Rhizoma Ligustici Wallichii (*Chuan Xiong*).

Also for lateral costal pain, add Rhizoma Corydalis Yanhusuo (*Yan Hu*) and Tuber Curcumae (*Yu Jin*).

If there is intercostal neuralgia, use Fructus Citri Seu Ponciri (*Zhi Ke*) instead of Citrus Immaturus and add Tuber Curcumae (*Yu Jin*), Bulbus Allii (*Xie Bai*), and Fructus Trichosanthis Kirlowii (*Gua Lou*).

For jaundice, add Herba Artemisiae Capillaris (*Yin Chen*), Fructus Gardeniae Jasminoidis (*Shan Zhi Zi*), and Tuber Curcumae (*Yu Jin*).

For chronic hepatitis with insomnia, excessive dreams, a bitter taste in the mouth, a red tongue with scant coating, and a wiry, thready, rapid pulse, add Herba Ecliptae Prostratae (*Han Lian Cao*), Fructus Ligustri Lucidi (*Nu Zhen Zi*), Concha Margaritiferae (*Zhen Zhu Mu*), and Radix Et Rhizoma Oryzae Glutinosae (*Nuo Dao Gen*).

For early cirrhosis of the liver with abdominal distention, bleeding gums, yellow urine, constipation, a red tongue with thin, yellow coating, and a wiry, thready, rapid pulse, add Radix Polygoni Multiflori (*He Shou Wu*), Herba Ecliptae Prostratae (*Han Lian Cao*), Carapax Amydae (*Bie Jia*), Concha Ostreae (*Mu Li*), and Fructus Meliae Toosendan (*Chuan Lian Zi*). If there is also edema and loose stools, add Rhizoma Atractylodis (*Cang Zhu*), Sclerotium Poriae Cocos (*Fu Ling*), and Squama Manitis (*Chuan Shan Jia*).

For biliary tract disorders, add Herba Artemisiae Capillaris (*Yin Chen*), Radix Salviae Miltiorrhizae (*Dan Shen*), Tuber Curcumae (*Yu Jin*), Radix Rubrus Paeoniae Lactiflorae (*Chi Shao*), and Herba Desmodii (*Jin Qian Cao*).

For acute biliary tract infection, add Herba Artemisiae Capillaris (*Yin Chen*), Tuber Curcumae (*Yu Jin*), Herba Andrographidis (*Chuan Xin Lian*), and Caulis In Taeniis Bambusae (*Zhu Ru*) to clear heat, eliminate dampness, and stop vomiting.

For chronic biliary tract infection, add Cortex Radicis Lycii (*Di Gu Pi*), Radix Et Rhizoma Oryzae Glutinosae (*Nuo Dao Gen*), Herba Dendrobii (*Shi Hu*), Radix Codonopsis Pilosulae (*Dang Shen*), and raw Concha Ostreae (*Sheng Mu Li*) to clear heat, enrich yin, and support the righteous.

For gallstones, add Herba Desmodii (*Jin Qian Cao*), Herba Artemisiae Capillaris (*Yin Chen*), and Endothelium Corneum Gigeriae Galli (*Ji Nei Jin*).

For biliary ascariasis, add Fructus Pruni Mume (*Wu Mei*) and Semen Arecae Catechu (*Bing Lang*).

Also for roundworms, add Fructus Pruni Mume (*Wu Mei*) and Cortex Radicis Meliae (*Ku Lian Gen Pi*).

For pain associated with blood stasis, add Radix Salviae Miltiorrhizae (*Dan Shen*) and Feces Trogopterori Seu Pteromi (*Wu Ling Zhi*) or Salvia and Radix Rubrus Paeoniae Lactiflorae (*Chi Shao*).

For food stagnation with abdominal pain, add Fructus Germinatus Hordei Vulgaris (*Mai Ya*), Fructus Crataegi (*Shan Zha*), and Endothelium Corneum Gigeriae Galli (*Ji Nei Jin*).

For irregular menstruation, replace Citrus Immaturus with Fructus Citri Seu Ponciri (*Zhi Ke*) and add Rhizoma Cyperi Rotundi (*Xiang Fu*), Rhizoma Ligustici Wallichii (*Chuan Xiong*), and Pericarpium Citri Reticulatae (*Chen Pi*).

For painful menstruation, add Radix Angelicae Sinensis (*Dang Gui*), Radix Linderae Strychnifoliae (*Wu Yao*), Rhizoma Cyperi Rotundi (*Xiang Fu*), and Rhizoma Corydalis Yanhusuo (*Yan Hu*).

For amenorrhea due to blood stasis, add Semen Pruni Persicae (*Tao Ren*) and Flos Carthami Tinctorii (*Hong Hua*).

For damp heat vaginal discharge with lower abdominal pain and soreness of the lower back, add *Er Miao San* (Two Wonders Powder).

For breast distention, add Pericarpium Viridis Citri Reticulatae (*Qing Pi*).

For acute mastitis, add Herba Cum Radice Taraxaci Mongolici (*Pu Gong Ying*), Herba Violae Yedoensis (*Zi Hua Di Ding*), and Flos Chrysanthemi Indici (*Ye Ju Hua*) to clear heat, resolve toxins, and disperse swelling.

For chronic mastitis, add Fructus Germinatus Hordei Vulgaris (*Mai Ya*) and Fructus Crataegi (*Shan Zha*) to disperse accumulation and stop milk production.

For fibrocystic lumps and mammary hyperplasia, add Squama Manitis (*Chuan Shan Jia*) and Semen Vaccariae Segetalis (*Wang Bu Liu Xing*) to dispel stasis, soften the hard, and scatter nodulation.

For intestinal obstruction, add Radix Et Rhizoma Rhei (*Da Huang*).

For acute icteric hepatitis, add *Yin Chen Hao Tang* (Artemisia Capillaris Decoction), *i.e.*, Herba Artemisiae Capillaris (*Yin Chen Hao*), Fructus Gardeniae Jasminoidis (*Zhi Zi*), and Radix et Rhizoma Rhei (*Da Huang*).

For facial flushing and headache, add Herba Menthae (*Bo He*) and Fructus Citri Seu Ponciri (*Zhi Ke*).

In case of severe diarrhea with tenesmus, add Bulbus Allii (*Xie Bai*).

For diarrhea with discharge of porridge-like stools, add Radix Saussureae Seu Vladimiriae (*Mu Xiang*) and Semen Arecae Catechu (*Bing Lang*).

For pediatric hernia, add Semen Litchi Sinensis (*Li Zhi He*).

For esophageal spasm, add Semen Oroxyli Indici (*Mu Hu Die*) and Fructus Germinatus Hordei Vulgaris (*Mai Ya*). In severe cases, add Radix Et Rhizoma Rhei (*Da Huang*).

For plum pit qi, replace Citrus Immaturus with Fructus Citri Seu Ponciri (*Zhi Ke*), subtract Licorice, and add processed Rhizoma Cyperi Rotundi (*Zhi Xiang Fu*), processed Rhizoma Pinelliae Ternatae (*Zhi Ban Xia*), Flos Pruni Mume (*Lu O Mei*), Caulis Perillae Frutescentis (*Su Geng*), Cortex Magnoliae Officinalis (*Hou Po*), raw Rhizoma Zingiberis (*Sheng Jiang*), and Fructus Zizyphi Jujubae (*Da Zao*).

Comment: In the pattern associated with this formula, although there are cold extremities, the red tongue and slightly rapid pulse indicate depressive heat is confined internally.

B. *Xiao Yao San* (Rambling Powder)

Composition:

Radix Bupleuri (*Chai Hu*), 9g
Radix Angelicae Sinensis (*Dang Gui*), 9g, slightly stir-fried
Radix Albus Paeoniae Lactiflorae (*Bai Shao*), 12g
Rhizoma Atractylodis Macrocephalae (*Bai Zhu*), 9g

Sclerotium Poriae Cocos (*Fu Ling*), 15g
Radix Glycyrrhizae (*Gan Cao*), 6g, mix-fried
Herba Menthae (*Bo He*), 3g
raw Rhizoma Zingiberis (*Sheng Jiang*), 3g

Functions: Courses the liver and resolves depression, fortifies the spleen and harmonizes the constructive

Indications: Liver depression, blood vacuity. Irregular menstruation, uterine bleeding, abnormal vaginal discharge, breast distention, premenstrual tension, climacteric disorders, chronic hepatitis, pleurisy, chronic gastritis, peptic ulcer, neurosis, anemia, insomnia, optic nerve atrophy, central retinitis, and neurasthenia.

Main signs & symptoms: Lateral coastal pain, alternating hot and cold, headache, vertigo, a dry mouth and throat, fatigued spirit, reduced appetite, menstrual irregularity, breast distention, a pale red tongue, and a wiry, fine, vacuous pulse.

Formula explanation:

In this formula, Bupleurum courses the liver and resolves depression. The combination of *Dang Gui* and Peony nourishes the blood and softens the liver. Because *Dang Gui* is somewhat aromatic, it moves the qi, but because it is sweet, it also relaxes tension. Therefore, it is an essential medicinal for treating liver depression with blood vacuity. Atractylodis and Poria fortify the spleen and remove dampness, thus promoting transportation and transformation and, ultimately, the origin of qi and blood. Mix-fried Licorice boosts the qi and supplements the center as well as relaxes the liver's tension. It is the assistant medicinal in this formula. The two messengers in this formula are Ginger and Mint. Ginger warms and harmonizes the center. Mint, when used in small amounts, assists Bupleurum's scattering of liver depression. Thus this formula as a whole regulates and harmonizes the liver and spleen.

Additions & subtractions:

If there is depressive heat, add Fructus Gardeniae Jasminoidis (*Shan Zhi Zi*) and Cortex Radicis Moutan (*Mu Dan Pi*). This results in *Dan Zhi Xiao Yao San* (Moutan & Gardenia Rambling Powder).

If there is more serious blood vacuity, add prepared Radix Rehmanniae (*Shu Di*). This results in *Hei Xiao Yao San* (Black Rambling Powder).

For concomitant qi vacuity, add Radix Panacis Ginseng (*Ren Shen*) or Radix Codonopsis Pilosulae (*Dang Shen*).

Also for qi vacuity, add Radix Codonopsis Pilosulae (*Dang Shen*) and Radix Pseudostellariae (*Tai Zi Shen*).

For qi vacuity and spleen weakness with borborygmus and loose stools, subtract Mint and add Radix Astragali Membranacei (*Huang Qi*), Rhizoma Cimicifugae (*Sheng Ma*), and mix-fried Radix Glycyrrhizae (*Zhi Gan Cao*).

For lateral costal pain, add Rhizoma Corydalis Yanhusuo (*Yan Hu*) and Fructus Meliae Toosendan (*Chuan Lian Zi*).

Also for lateral costal pain, subtract Atractylodis and add Rhizoma Cyperi Rotundi (*Xiang Fu*).

For intense, fixed pain due to blood stasis, add Cortex Radicis Moutan (*Dan Pi*), Tuber Curcumae (*Yu Jin*), and Rhizoma Sparganii (*San Leng*).

For cold hernia pain due to cold and dampness attacking the small intestine, subtract Peony, Mint, and Bupleurum and add Fructus Meliae Toosendan (*Chuan Lian Zi*), Fructus Evodiae Rutecarpae (*Wu

Zhu Yu), Radix Saussureae Seu Vladimiriae (*Mu Xiang*), and Fructus Foeniculi Vulgaris (*Xiao Hui Xiang*).

For abnormal vaginal discharge, add Flos Lonicerae Japonicae (*Yin Hua*) and Rhizoma Dryopteridis Seu Blechni (*Guan Zhong*).

Also for abnormal vaginal discharge, add Rhizoma Dioscoreae Hypoglaucae (*Bi Xie*), Semen Plantaginis (*Che Qian Zi*), and Cortex Cedrelae (*Chun Pi*).

If abnormal vaginal discharge is due to downward percolation of spleen/kidney damp heat, add Radix Dioscoreae Oppositae (*Shan Yao*), Semen Euryalis Ferocis (*Qian Shi*), and Semen Plantaginis (*Che Qian Zi*).

For vaginal itching and burning urination, add Radix Gentianae Scabrae (*Long Dan Cao*), Fructus Gardeniae Jasminoidis (*Zhi Zi*), Radix Scutellariae Baicalensis (*Huang Qin*), Rhizoma Alismatis (*Ze Xie*), and Caulis Akebiae Mutong (*Mu Tong*).

For pain in the area of the liver with reduced appetite and fatigue, subtract Ginger and Mint and add Rhizoma Cyperi Rotundi (*Xiang Fu*), Fructus Citri Sacrodactylis (*Fo Shou*), Radix Salviae Miltior-rhizae (*Dan Shen*), and Radix Codonopsis Pilosulae (*Dang Shen*).

For an enlarged liver and spleen, add Os Sepiae Seu Sepiellae (*Wu Zei Gu*), Carapax Amydae (*Bie Jia*), and Concha Ostreae (*Mu Li*).

For an enlarged, hard liver with a dull, black facial color and cyanotic lips, add Rhizoma Sparganii (*San Leng*), Rhizoma Curcumae Zedoariae (*E Zhu*), Flos Carthami Tinctorii (*Hong Hua*), and Radix Salviae Miltiorrhizae (*Dan Shen*).

49

For fibrocystic breasts, subtract Licorice and add Semen Vaccariae Segetalis (*Wang Bu Liu Xing*), Caulis Millettiae Seu Spatholobi (*Ji Xue Teng*), Radix Salviae Miltiorrhizae (*Dan Shen*), and Rhizoma Cyperi Rotundi (*Xiang Fu*).

For premenstrual breast distention and pain, add Fructus Trichosanthis Kirlowii (*Gua Lou*) and Radix Et Rhizoma Notopterygii (*Qiang Huo*).

For hypertension, add Spica Prunellae Vulgaris (*Xia Gu Cao*), Ramus Loranthi Seu Visci (*Sang Ji Sheng*), and Fructus Ligustri Lucidi (*Nu Zhen Zi*).

For various ophthalmological disorders, such as glaucoma, optic nerve atrophy, acute retrobulbar neuritis, cortical blindness, and central retinitis, add Flos Chrysanthemi Morifolii (*Ju Hua*), Fructus Lycii Chinensis (*Gou Qi Zi*), and Rhizoma Acori Graminei (*Shi Chang Pu*).

For red eyes and mental dullness due to upward rising of depressive heat of the heart, liver, and spleen, add Rhizoma Ligustici Wallichii (*Chuan Xiong*), Flos Chrysanthemi Morifolii (*Ju Hua*), Flos Lonicerae Japonicae (*Yin Hua*), Radix Scutellariae Baicalensis (*Huang Qin*), and Rhizoma Coptidis Chinensis (*Huang Lian*).

For insomnia, add Concha Ostreae (*Mu Li*) and Os Draconis (*Long Gu*).

For insomnia and excessive dreams, add Semen Zizyphi Spinosae (*Suan Zao Ren*) and Semen Biotae Orientalis (*Bai Zi Ren*).

For insomnia, excessive dreams, mental dullness, and vertigo, add *Suan Zao Ren Tang* (Zizyphus Spinosa Decoction), *i.e.*, Semen Zizyphi Spinosae (*Suan Zao Ren*), Sclerotium Poriae Cocos (*Fu Ling*), Rhizoma Ligustici Wallichii (*Chuan Xiong*), Rhizoma Anemarrhena (*Zhi Mu*), and Radix Glycyrrhizae (*Gan Cao*).

50

For abdominal distention, add Cortex Magnoliae Officinalis (*Hou Po*) and Pericarpium Citri Reticulatae (*Chen Pi*).

For abdominal distention and decreased food intake, add Rhizoma Pinelliae Ternatae (*Ban Xia*), Fructus Cardamomi (*Bai Dou Kou*), and Fructus Germinatus Hordei Vulgaris (*Mai Ya*).

For abdominal distention, fatigue, and decreased food intake, add Radix Codonopsis Pilosulae (*Dang Shen*), Fructus Germinatus Hordei Vulgaris (*Mai Ya*), and Endothelium Corneum Gigeriae Galli (*Ji Nei Jin*).

For abdominal distention, loose stools, borborygmus, and flatulence, add *Xiang Sha Liu Jun Zi Tang* (Saussurea & Amomum Six Gentlemen Decoction), *i.e.*, Radix Panacis Ginseng (*Ren Shen*), Rhizoma Atractylodis Macrocephalae (*Bai Zhu*), Sclerotium Poriae Cocos (*Fu Ling*), mix-fried Radix Glycyrrhizae (*Zhi Gan Cao*), Rhizoma Pinelliae Ternatae (*Ban Xia*), Pericarpium Citri Reticulatae (*Chen Pi*), Fructus Amomi (*Sha Ren*), and Radix Saussureae Seu Vladimiriae (*Mu Xiang*).

For acne, use *Dan Zhi Xiao Yao San* and add Fructus Arctii Lappae (*Niu Bang Zi*) and Fructus Forsythiae Suspensae (*Lian Qiao*).

For diarrhea, add Rhizoma Pinelliae Ternatae (*Ban Xia*) and Radix Dioscoreae Oppositae (*Shan Yao*).

If there is headache accompanying the period, add Herba Seu Flos Schizonepetae Tenuifoliae (*Jing Jie*) and Radix Angelicae (*Bai Zhi*).

If there is nervous excitability, add Rhizoma Ligustici Wallichii (*Chuan Xiong*) and Ramulus Uncariae Cum Uncis (*Gou Teng*).

For nervous anxiety and agitation due to liver qi disturbing the heart spirit, add Cinnabaris (*Zhu Sha*) and Radix Polygalae Tenuifoliae (*Yuan Zhi*).

For yin vacuity with a red tongue and scant coating, add Fructus Ligustri Lucidi (*Nu Zhen Zi*), Herba Ecliptae Prostratae (*Han Lian Cao*), and Fructus Lycii Chinensis (*Gou Qi Zi*).

For edema of the lower extremities and scanty urination, add Herba Dianthi (*Qu Mai*), Herba Polygoni Avicularis (*Bian Xu*), Rhizoma Alismatis (*Ze Xie*), and Semen Plantaginis (*Che Qian Zi*).

For nosebleeding and bleeding gums, add raw Radix Rehmanniae (*Sheng Di*), Cortex Radicis Moutan (*Dan Pi*), and Rhizoma Imperatae Cylindricae (*Bai Mao Gen*).

If there is nosebleeding due to depressive heat of the heart, lung, and liver, add Radix Rubiae Cordifoliae (*Qian Cao*).

For premenstrual nosebleeding, add carbonized Fructus Gardeniae Jasminoidis (*Shan Zhi Tan*), Rhizoma Imperatae Cylindricae (*Bai Mao Gen*), Herba Cephalanoplos (*Xiao Ji*), and Radix Cyathulae (*Chuan Niu Xi*).

For dry mouth and thirst, add raw Radix Rehmanniae (*Sheng Di*) and Radix Trichosanthis Kirlowii (*Tian Hua Fen*).

For headache and vertigo, add Rhizoma Gastrodiae Elatae (*Tian Ma*), Ramulus Uncariae Cum Uncis (*Gou Teng*), and Flos Chrysanthemi Morifolii (*Ju Hua*).

If there is a flushed face, heart vexation, and easy anger, to *Dan Zhi Xiao Yao San* add Rhizoma Coptidis Chinensis (*Huang Lian*) and Radix Gentianae Scabrae (*Long Dan Cao*).

For internal confinement of damp heat with jaundice, add Cortex Phellodendri (*Huang Bai*), Herba Artemisiae Capillaris (*Yin Chen*), and Fructus Gardeniae Jasminoidis (*Zhi Zi*).

For flooding (*i.e.*, uterine bleeding) due to anger damaging the liver or continuous, purple-colored spotting with clots, lower abdominal distention, fullness and oppression of the chest and upper abdomen, shortness of breath, decreased food intake, fatigue, and indigestion, subtract *Dang Gui* and Licorice and add Radix Adenophorae Strictae (*Nan Sha Shen*), stir-fried Pollen Typhae (*Chao Pu Huang*), Crinis Carbonisatus (*Xue Yu Tan*), and blackened Folium Artemisiae Argyii (*Hei Ai Ye*). This results in *Fu Pi Shu Gan Tang* (Support the Spleen, Soothe the Liver Decoction).

For continuous bleeding and spotting with distention and pain in the lower abdomen, add Radix Scutellariae Baicalensis (*Huang Qin*) and Cortex Phellodendri (*Huang Bai*).

For bleeding during pregnancy due to depressive heat and stasis, subtract *Dang Gui* and Licorice and add Fructus Gardeniae Jasminoidis (*Zhi Zi*) and Herba Leonuri Heterophylli (*Yi Mu Cao*). This results in *Shu Yu Qing Gan Yin* (Soothe Depression, Clear the Liver Drink).

For hot strangury, to *Dan Zhi Xiao Yao San* add Semen Plantaginis (*Che Qian Zi*).

For early, late, or erratic periods with distention and pain and the sensation of heat in the lower abdomen, add Rhizoma Cyperi Rotundi (*Xiang Fu*), Tuber Curcumae (*Yu Jin*), and Herba Seu Flos Schizonepetae Tenuifoliae (*Jing Jie Sui*).

For early periods with a heavy, red discharge, add raw Radix Rehmanniae (*Sheng Di*) and Carapax Amydae (*Bie Jia*).

For scanty menstruation with purplish clots and abdominal pain, add Rhizoma Ligustici Wallichii (*Chuan Xiong*) and Tuber Curcumae (*Yu Jin*).

For perimenstrual numbness of the extremities with yang vacuity and weak qi, add Ramulus Cinnamomi (*Gui Zhi*) and Exocarpium Citri Rubri (*Ju Hong*).

For perimenstrual edema due to earth not generating metal with non-diffusion of lung qi, add Cortex Cinnamomi (*Rou Gui*) and Radix Glehniae Littoralis (*Bei Sha Shen*).

For women with liver depression, qi stagnation and cough and vomiting due to phlegm dampness attacking the lungs and stomach, add Exocarpium Citri Rubri (*Ju Hong*), Bulbus Fritillariae (*Bei Mu*), and Rhizoma Pinelliae Ternatae (*Ban Xia*).

For women with constipation due to heat in the stomach and intestines, add Radix Et Rhizoma Rhei (*Da Huang*) and Mirabilitum (*Mang Xiao*).

For galactorrhea, add Radix Albus Paeoniae Lactiflorae (*Bai Shao*) and stir-fried Fructus Germinatus Hordei Vulgaris (*Chao Mai Ya*).

Comment: This is one of the most commonly used formulas in Chinese medicine. It is especially useful in the treatment of various gynecological complaints.

3.3 *Tiao He Chang Wei Ji* (Regulating & harmonizing the intestines & stomach formulas)

Representative formula: *Ban Xia Xie Xin Tang* (Pinellia Drain the Heart Decoction)

Composition:

Rhizoma Pinelliae Ternatae (*Ban Xia*), 9g
Radix Scutellariae Baicalensis (*Huang Qin*), 9g
dry Rhizoma Zingiberis (*Gan Jiang*), 6g
Radix Panacis Ginseng (*Ren Shen*), 9g
Radix Glycyrrhizae (*Gan Cao*), 6g, mix-fried
Rhizoma Coptidis Chinensis (*Huang Lian*), 3g
Fructus Zizyphi Jujubae (*Da Zao*), 4 pieces

Functions: Harmonizes the stomach and downbears counterflow, opens binding and eliminates glomus

Indications: Lack of harmony of the stomach. Acute and chronic gastritis, enteritis, indigestion, pediatric vomiting and diarrhea, chronic hepatitis, early-stage cirrhosis, and gastric ulcers due to hyperacidity

Main signs & symptoms: Glomus and fullness below the heart but no pain, vomiting or dry heaves, borborygmus, diarrhea, a thin, yellow or slimy tongue coating, and wiry, rapid pulse

Formula explanation:

This formula is a modification of *Xiao Chai Hu Tang*. It is used when there is diarrhea and detriment damage of the central yang with possible external evils obstructing the (qi) dynamic. In this case, cold and heat are mutually binding, producing glomus underneath the heart since the qi is not upbearing and downbearing, is full and not free

55

flowing. Coptis and Scutellaria are bitter and cold, downbearing and discharging. Thus they eliminate heat. Dry Ginger and Pinellia are acrid, warm, and open nodulation, thus scattering cold. Ginseng, Licorice, and Red Dates are sweet and warm and boost the qi, thus supplementing vacuity. When these 7 flavors (*i.e.*, ingredients) are combined, cold and hot (medicinals) are used together as are bitter, downbearing and acrid, opening ingredients. In addition, the qi is supplemented and the center is harmonized. Therefore, evils are removed at the same time as the righteous is augmented.

Additions & subtractions:

For damp heat accumulating in the middle burner with vomiting, glomus, and fullness, subtract Ginseng, dry Ginger, Red Dates and mix-fried Licorice and add Fructus Immaturus Citri Seu Ponciri (*Zhi Shi*) and raw Rhizoma Zingiberis (*Sheng Jiang*).

For more serious stomach qi vacuity with undigested food in the stool and irritability, increase the dosage of mix-fried Licorice to 12-15g. This results in *Gan Cao Xie Xin Tang* (Licorice Drain the Heart Decoction).

For water and heat struggling in the middle burner or for stomach vacuity with food stagnation, replace dry Ginger with raw Rhizoma Zingiberis (*Sheng Jiang*). This results in *Sheng Jiang Xie Xin Tang* (Fresh Ginger Drain the Heart Decoction).

For heat in the chest and cold in the stomach with chest oppression and irritability, nausea, abdominal pain, a white, slimy tongue coating, and wiry pulse, subtract Scutellaria and add Ramulus Cinnamomi (*Gui Zhi*). This results in *Huang Lian Tang* (Coptis Decoction).

For abdominal pain, add Fructus Amomi (*Sha Ren*) and Radix Saussureae Seu Vladimiriae (*Mu Xiang*).

For chronic diarrhea, add Radix Puerariae Lobatae (*Ge Gen*).

For plum pit qi, add Cortex Magnoliae Officinalis (*Hou Po*).

For chest oppression and distention, add Radix Bupleuri (*Chai Hu*) and Semen Trichosanthis Kirlowii (*Gua Lou Ren*). This results in *Chai Xian Tang* (Bupleurum Fall Decoction).

Comment: This formula can be used without the presence of any external evils. Heat can be transformative heat and cold may simply be due to exuberant yin and insufficient yang.

銀翹散主上焦醫
竹葉荊牛薄荷枝
甘桔蘆根涼解法
風溫初感此方宜
咳加杏貝渴花粉
熱甚梔苓次第施

Mnemonic verse for learning *Yin Qiao San*

4

Qing Re Ji
Clearing Heat Formulas

Formulas in this category are mainly composed of heat-clearing medicinals. They clear heat, drain fire, cool the blood, resolve toxins, and enrich yin. Heat-clearing formulas are used to clear internal heat where there is neither an external pattern nor internal accumulation and binding. When prescribing heat-clearing formulas, one must clearly distinguish whether the heat is replete or vacuous and also where the heat is located. Location in this context means either a) the *fen* or division *vis á vis wen bing xue* or warm disease theory or b) the viscera and bowels.

There are six subcategories of heat-clearing formulas. These are 1) formulas which cleat heat from the *qi fen* or division, 2) formulas which clear the constructive and cool the blood, 3) formulas which clear heat and resolve toxins, 4) formulas which clear heat and dispel summerheat, 5) formulas which clear heat from the viscera and bowels, and 6) formulas which clear vacuity heat. Within warm disease theory, heat in the qi division is essentially the same as a *yang ming* division disorder in the *Shang Han Lun (Treatise on Damage by Cold)*. Toxins refer to especially dense concentrations of evils which have become bound or knotted. Under the clearing heat from the viscera and bowels subcategory, there are various formulas which clear heat from specific viscera and specific bowels.

Cautions & Contraindications When Using Heat-clearing Formulas

1. Because these formulas are mostly composed of bitter, cold medicinals, their excessive or prolonged use can damage the spleen/stomach. Therefore, they should be used only when necessary and their use should be discontinued as soon as the evil heat is cleared.
2. Based on the above, in some cases it is necessary to include ingredients which protect the stomach qi and yin when using bitter, cold medicinals.

4.1 *Qing Qi Fen Ji* (Formulas for clearing heat from the qi division)

Representative formula: *Bai Hu Tang* (White Tiger Decoction)

Composition:

Gypsum (*Shi Gao*), 30g
Rhizoma Anemarrhenae (*Zhi Mu*), 9g
Radix Glycyrrhizae (*Gan Cao*), 3g, mix-fried
Semen Oryzae Sativae (*Jing Mi*), 9g

Functions: Clears heat and engenders fluids

Indications: *Yang ming* qi division exuberance of heat. Gingivitis, encephalitis B, epidemic meningitis, diabetes mellitus, lobar pneumonia, high fever due to febrile disease, erysipelas, scarlatina, measles, common cold, flus, anxiety and emotional disorders, eczema, and pruritus

Main signs & symptoms: High fever, red face, vexatious thirst and a desire for cold drinks, sweating, aversion to heat, possible headache, toothache, nosebleed, or bleeding gums, a flooding, large, forceful or slippery, rapid pulse

Contraindications:

1. Do not use for fever due to spleen/stomach vacuity, in which case rootless yang qi floats upward and outward to the exterior.
2. Do not use for false heat/true cold.

Formula explanation:

Within this formula, Gypsum is the sovereign. Gypsum is acrid, sweet, and greatly cold. It controls exuberant internal heat in the *yang ming*. Anemarrhena is the minister medicinal. It is bitter, cold, and moist in nature. It assists Gypsum in clearing heat from the lungs and stomach. Since it is bitter and cold and moistens dryness, it also enriches yin. Licorice and Rice are able to boost the stomach and protect fluids. These are the assistants.

Additions & subtractions:

For concomitant qi vacuity as evidenced by a large, forceless pulse, add Radix Panacis Ginseng (*Ren Shen*). This results in *Ren Shen Bai Hu Tang* (Ginseng White Tiger Decoction).

For swelling of the joints due to wind, damp, heat *bi*, add Rhizoma Atractylodis (*Cang Zhu*). This results in *Bai Hu Jia Cang Zhu Tang* (White Tiger Plus Atractylodis Decoction).

For pain in the joints due to wind, damp, heat painful *bi*, add Ramulus Cinnamomi (*Gui Zhi*). This results in *Bai Hu Jia Gui Zhi Tang* (White Tiger Plus Cinnamon Decoction).

For high fever with irritability, loss of consciousness of human affairs, and convulsions, add Cornu Antelopis (*Ling Yang Jiao*) and Cornu Rhinocerotis (*Xi Jiao*). This results in *Ling Xi Bai Hu Tang* (Antelope & Rhinoceros White Tiger Decoction).

For convulsions and spasms due to high fever, add Cornu Antelopis (*Ling Yang Jiao*), Lumbricus (*Di Long*), and Ramulus Uncariae Cum Uncis (*Gou Teng*).

For high fever and constipation with excessive sweating, thirst, irritability, reddish yellow, scanty, painful urination, and, in severe cases, delirious speech or mania, add Radix Et Rhizoma Rhei (*Da Huang*). This results in *Bai Hu Cheng Qi Tang* (White Tiger Order the Qi Decoction).

For severe fever alternating with mild chills due to simultaneous *yang ming/shao yang* pattern, add Radix Bupleurum (*Chai Hu*), Radix Scutellariae Baicalensis (*Huang Qin*), Radix Trichosanthis Kirlowii (*Tian Hua Fen*), and Folium Nelumbinis Nuciferae (*Xian He Ye*). This results in *Chai Hu Bai Hu Tang* (Bupleurum White Tiger Decoction).

For nausea, add Caulis In Taeniis Bambusae (*Zhu Ru*).

For *yang ming* symptoms with counterflow stomach qi, subtract Licorice and Rice and add Rhizoma Pinelliae Ternatae (*Ban Xia*) and Caulis In Taeniis Bambusae (*Zhu Ru*). This results in *Zhen Ni Bai Hu Tang* (Suppress Counterflow White Tiger Decoction).

For encephalitis and meningitis, add Flos Lonicerae Japonicae (*Yin Hua*) and Fructus Forsythiae Suspensae (*Lian Qiao*).

For excessive phlegm, add Radix Platycodi Grandiflori (*Jie Geng*).

For acute upper respiratory tract infection with bodily weakness and vacuity, subtract Anemarrhena and add Radix Panacis Ginseng (*Ren Shen*), Folium Bambusae (*Zhu Ye*), Tuber Ophiopogonis Japonicae (*Mai Dong*), and Rhizoma Pinelliae Ternatae (*Ban Xia*). This results in *Zhu Ye Shi Gao Tang* (Bamboo Leaf & Gypsum Decoction).

For diabetes with polydipsia and polyphagia, add Radix Trichosanthis Kirlowii (*Tian Hua Fen*).

4.2 *Qing Ying Liang Xue Ji* (Formulas for clearing the constructive & cooling the blood)

Representative formula: *Xi Jiao Di Huang Tang* (Rhinoceros & Rehmannia Decoction)

Composition:

Cornu Rhinocerotis (*Xi Jiao*), 3g
raw Radix Rehmanniae (*Sheng Di*), 30g
Radix Rubrus Paeoniae Lactiflorae (*Chi Shao*), 12g
Cortex Radicis Moutan (*Mu Dan Pi*), 9g

Functions: Clears heat and resolves toxins, cools the blood and scatters stasis

Indications: 1) Heat damaging the blood network vessels, 2) amassed blood, retained stasis, 3) heat harassing the heart constructive. Various sorts of hemorrhage, infectious febrile diseases with hemorrhage, measles, septicemia, encephalitis, meningitis, toxemia, uremia, hepatic coma, thrombocytopenic purpura, blood or pus in the anterior chamber of the eye, iridocyclitis, glaucoma, acute leukemia, mental illness, and burns

Main signs & symptoms: 1) Vomiting blood, hacking up blood, bloody stools, and other such hemorrhagic conditions; 2) mania, thirst with inability to swallow, vexatious pain inside the chest, abdominal distention; 3) mania and delirious speech, blackish purple petechiae, a scarlet tongue with prickles, and a thready, rapid pulse

Contraindications:

1. Do not use for bleeding due to yang vacuity or spleen qi vacuity.

Formula explanation:

In this formula, Rhinoceros Horn clears the heart, cools the blood, and resolves toxins and is the ruler. Combined with raw Rehmannia, they cool the blood and stop bleeding while nourishing the blood and clearing heat. Red Peony and Moutan are able to cool the blood and also scatter stasis. Thus this formula not only cools the blood but also quickens the blood and scatters stasis.

Additions & subtractions:

For manic behavior, add Radix Scutellariae Baicalensis (*Huang Qin*) and Radix Et Rhizoma Rhei (*Da Huang*).

For hematemesis and epistaxis, add Cacumen Biotae Orientalis (*Ce Bai Ye*), Rhizoma Imperatae Cylindricae (*Bai Mao Gen*), and Herba Ecliptae Prostratae (*Han Lian Cao*).

For hemafecia, add Radix Sanguisorbae (*Di Yu*) and Flos Immaturus Sophorae Japonicae (*Huai Hua*).

For hematuria, add Rhizoma Imperatae Cylindricae (*Bai Mao Gen*) and Herba Cephalanoplos (*Xiao Ji*).

For severe damage of the yin and blood, replace Red Peony with Radix Albus Paeoniae Lactiflorae (*Bai Shao*).

For easy anger due to liver depression, add Radix Bupleuri (*Chai Hu*), Radix Scutellariae Baicalensis (*Huang Qin*), and Fructus Gardeniae Jasminoidis (*Zhi Zi*).

For rashes, add Radix Lithospermi Seu Arnebiae (*Zi Cao*) and Pulvis Indigonis (*Qing Dai*).

For severe bleeding, add Pulvis Radicis Pseudoginseng (*San Qi Fen*).

For high fever and loss of consciousness of human affairs, add *An Gong Niu Huang Wan* (Quiet the Palace Bezoar Pills). See portal-opening formulas for ingredients.

For heat entering the blood division complicated by stasis, add Semen Pruni Persicae (*Tao Ren*) and Flos Campsitis (*Ling Xiao Hua*).

Comment: Cornu Bubali (*Shui Niu Jiao*) can be substituted for Rhinoceros Horn. In either case, the horn is ground into a fine powder and washed down with the decoction. It is also possible to substitute Radix Lithospermi Seu Arnebiae (*Zi Cao*) for Rhinoceros Horn. One may also substitute Gypsum (*Shi Gao*) and Radix Isatidis Seu Baphicacanthi (*Ban Lan Gen*). Since Rhinoceros are an endangered species, such substitution is imperative.

4.3 *Qing Re Jie Du Ji* (Formulas for clearing heat & resolving toxins)

Representative formula: *Huang Lian Jie Du Tang* (Coptis Resolve Toxins Decoction)

Composition:

Rhizoma Coptidis (*Huang Lian*), 3-9g

Radix Scutellariae Baicalensis (*Huang Qin*), 6g
Cortex Phellodendri (*Huang Bai*), 6g
Fructus Gardeniae Jasminoidis (*Zhi Zi*), 9g

Functions: Drains fire and resolves toxins

Indications: Replete heat and fire toxins, exuberant heat in the three burners patterns. Septicemia, dysentery, pneumonia, acute urinary tract infections, ulcers, carbuncles, furuncles, boils, acute enteritis, acute icteric hepatitis, acute cholecystitis, encephalitis, acute conjunctivitis, acute pelvic inflammation, erysipelas, cellulitis, hemoptysis, epistaxis, urticaria, pruritus, cerebral hemorrhage, hypertension, anxiety, palpitations, insomnia, neurasthenia, and hysteria

Main signs & symptoms: Great heat, vexation and agitation, a dry mouth and throat, delirious speech, insomnia, possible hot diseases with hemoptysis and/or epistaxis, possible high fever with macular eruptions, generalized heat with dysentery, damp heat jaundice, a red tongue with yellow coating, and a fast, forceful pulse

Contraindications:

1. Do not use in patients with bodily vacuity or weakness of the spleen and stomach.
2. Do not administer for prolonged periods of time.
3. Do not use for heat in the constructive or blood levels.

Formula explanation:

In this formula, Coptis is the sovereign. It drains heart fire as well as draining fire from the middle burner. Scutellaria clears lung heat and drains upper burner fire. It acts as the minister. Phellodendron and Gardenia are the assistants. Phellodendron drains fire from the lower burner and Gardenia opens and drains fire from all three burners. It leads heat downward and moves it. Therefore, as a whole, this formula has the functions of draining fire, clearing heat, and resolving toxins.

Additions & subtractions:

If there is constipation, add Radix Et Rhizoma Rhei (*Da Huang*) to drain and precipitate replete heat.

If there is hematemesis, epistasis, and macular eruptions, add raw Radix Rehmanniae (*Sheng Di*), Radix Scrophulariae Ningpoensis (*Yuan Shen*), and Cortex Radicis Moutan (*Dan Pi*) to cool the blood and transform maculae, clear heat and stop bleeding.

Or take with *Xi Jiao Di Huang Tang* (Rhinoceros Horn & Rehmannia Decoction). See above.

Or add Rhizoma Imperatae Cylindricae (*Bai Mao Gen*) and Cacumen Biotae Orientalis (*Ce Bai Ye*).

For severe maculae, add Cortex Radicis Moutan (*Dan Pi*) and raw Radix Rehmanniae (*Sheng Di*).

If there is stasis heat with jaundice, add Herba Artemisiae Capillaris (*Yin Chen*) and Radix Et Rhizoma Rhei (*Da Huang*) in order to strengthen the clearing of heat and resolving of toxins, the elimination of dampness and receding of yellowing.

For delirious speech and constipation, add *Cheng Qi Tang* (Order the Qi Decoction). But if there is delirious speech and the bowels are open and uninhibited, simply take *Si Wei Huang Lian Chu Re Tang* (Four Flavors Coptis Eliminate Heat Decoction), *i.e.*, *Huang Lian Jie Du Tang* as above.

For damp heat in the lower burner with frequent urination, urgency, and pain, add Caulis Akebiae Mutong (*Mu Tong*), Rhizoma Alismatis (*Ze Xie*), and Semen Plantaginis (*Che Qian Zi*).

For red and white dysentery (*i.e.*, for dysentery with pus and blood) and tenesmus, add Radix Saussureae Seu Vladimiriae (*Mu Xiang*), Semen Arecae Catechu (*Bing Lang*), and Cortex Fraxini (*Qin Pi*).

For toxic lesions, such as deep-rooted boils, add *Wu Wei Xiao Du Yin* (Five Flavors Disperse Toxins Drink), *i.e.*, Flos Lonicerae Japonicae (*Yin Hua*), Herba Cum Radice Taraxaci Mongolici (*Pu Gong Ying*), Flos Chrysanthemi Indici (*Ye Ju Hua*), Herba Cum Radice Violae Yedoensis (*Zi Hua Di Ding*), Herba Begoniae Fimbristipulatae (*Ze Bei Tian Kuei*).

If there is a red tongue with no coating, add Radix Scrophulariae Ningpoensis (*Yuan Shen*), raw Radix Rehmanniae (*Sheng Di*), and Tuber Ophiopogonis Japonicae (*Mai Dong*).

If there is concomitant yin vacuity, add prepared Radix Rehmanniae (*Shu Di*) and Rhizoma Anemarrhenae (*Zhi Mu*).

If there is concomitant blood vacuity, add *Si Wu Tang* (Four Materials Decoction), *i.e.*, Radix Angelicae Sinensis (*Dang Gui*), Radix Albus Paeoniae Lactiflorae (*Bai Shao*), prepared Radix Rehmannia (*Shu Di*), and Rhizoma Ligustici Wallichii (*Chuan Xiong*). This results in *Wen Qing Yin* (Warm & Clear Drink).

For insomnia, add Semen Zizyphi Spinosae (*Suan Zao Ren*).

For hot diarrhea and dysentery, add Radix Puerariae Lobatae (*Ge Gen*).

For acne rosacea, add Flos Carthami Tinctorii (*Hong Hua*), raw Radix Rehmanniae (*Sheng Di*), and Radix Rubrus Paeoniae Lactiflorae (*Chi Shao*).

For oral ulcers and cold sores, add Herba Menthae (*Bo He*) and Fructus Forsythiae Suspensae (*Lian Qiao*).

For heartburn, add Concha Ostreae (*Mu Li*).

For boils, ear infection, or conjunctivitis, add Radix Ledebouriellae Sesloidis (*Fang Feng*), Herba Menthae (*Bo He*), Herba Seu Flos Schizonepetae Tenuifoliae (*Jing Jie Sui*), and Fructus Forsythiae Suspensae (*Lian Qiao*).

For extreme thirst, facial flushing or rash, and a large pulse, add Gypsum (*Shi Gao*), Herba Ephedrae (*Ma Huang*), Semen Praeparatus Sojae (*Dan Dou Chi*), and raw Rhizoma Zingiberis (*Sheng Jiang*). This results in *San Huang Shi Gao Tang* (Three Yellows Gypsum Decoction) minus Red Dates and Tea.

For high fever and jaundice, add Radix Et Rhizoma Rhei (*Da Huang*) and Herba Artemisiae Capillaris (*Yin Chen*).

Comment: This formula is composed of TCM's most often used anti-mycotic, antibacterial ingredients. For serious conditions, one needs to either add ingredients or increase its dosages. This formula can be used simultaneously with antibiotics administered either orally or intravenously. For use against sores and boils, such sores should be treated locally with external applications as well as internally (*i.e.*, systemically).

4.4 *Qing Re Zhu Shu Ji* (Formulas for clearing heat & dispelling summerheat)

Representative formula: *Liu Yi San* (Six to One Powder)

Composition:

Talcum (*Hua Shi*)
Radix Glycyrrhizae (*Gan Cao*)

Method of preparation & administration: Grind 6 parts Talcum to 1 part Licorice and take 9-18g each time with warm water. These ingredients may also be decocted, in which case Talcum should be placed in a fine cloth bag.

Functions: Dispels summerheat and disinhibits dampness

Indications: External invasion of summerheat dampness. Upper respiratory tract infection, urinary tract infection, and acute gastroenteritis

Main signs & symptoms: High fever, vexation and agitation, thirst, inhibited,astringent urination, vomiting or diarrhea, a thin, slimy tongue coating, and a forceful, rapid pulse

Contraindications:

1. Do not use with the elderly, those with bodily vacuity weakness, or those with yin vacuity since it may easily damage qi and fluids.
2. Do not use in cases with copious, clear urine or in cases of sum merheat without concomitant dampness.

Formula explanation:

In this formula, cold, bland Talcum clears heat and disinhibits urination. It is the sovereign ingredient in *Liu Yi San*. Licorice is Talcum's minister. It harmonizes the middle burner. If used raw, it also clears heat and resolves toxins. However, because Licorice is sweet, it generates fluids and therefore protects against fluid damage by Talcum's promotion of diuresis.

Additions & subtractions:

For urinary strangury, including pain and stones, add Spora Lygodii (*Hai Jin Sha*), Herba Desmodii (*Jin Qian Cao*), and Endothelium Corneum Gigeriae Galli (*Ji Nei Jin*).

For strong summerheat with excessive thirst, irritability, and scanty, reddish yellow urination, add Pericarpium Citrulli Vulgaris (*Xi Gua Pi*) or Fructus Citrulli Vulgaris prepared with Mirabilitum (*Xi Gua Shuang*), Fasciculus Vascularis Luffae (*Si Gua Luo*), and Folium Bambusae (*Zhu Ye*).

For hematuria, pain, frequency, and urgency, add Rhizoma Imperatae Cylindricae (*Bai Mao Gen*), Herba Cephalanoplos (*Xiao Ji*), Herba Cirsii (*Da Ji*), and Cacumen Biotae Orientalis (*Ce Bai Ye*).

For red yes, sore throat, or ulceration of the mouth and tongue, add Pulvis Indigonis (*Qing Dai*). This results in *Bi Yu San* (Green Jade Powder).

If there are fever and aversion to cold due to exterior patterns of summerheat and dampness, add Herba Menthae (*Bo He*). This results in *Ji Su San* (Cock-waking Powder).

For summerheat patterns with irritability, add Cinnabaris (*Zhu Sha*) and take with a decoction of Medulla Junci Effusi (*Deng Xin Cao*). This results in *Yi Yuan San* (Boost the Source Powder).

For dry summerheat, replace Talcum with Gypsum (*Shi Gao*).

For severe thirst with a red tongue, add Tuber Ophiopogonis Japonicae (*Mai Dong*), Radix Glehniae Littoralis (*Sha Shen*), Herba Dendrobii (*Shi Hu*), and Rhizoma Anemarrhenae (*Zhi Mu*).

For damage to qi and body fluids, add Radix Panacis Quinquefolii (*Xi Yang Shen*).

For cystitis or urethritis, add Cortex Phellodendri (*Huang Bai*).

Comments: This formula is rarely used alone. Usually it is added to other formulas in order to clear heat and disinhibit dampness.

4.5 *Qing Zang Fu Re Ji* (Formulas for clearing heat from the viscera & bowels)

Representative formulas:

A. *Dao Chi San* (Lead [Out] the Red Powder)

Composition:

raw Radix Rehmanniae (*Sheng Di*), 15g
Caulis Akebiae Mutong (*Mu Tong*), 12g
raw Radix Glycyrrhizae (*Sheng Gan Cao Xiao*), 6g
Folium Bambusae (*Zhu Ye*), 9g

Functions: Clears the heart and nourishes yin, disinhibits water and opens strangury

Indications: Heart fire affecting the small intestine and bladder. Acute cystitis, urethritis, difficult urination, glomerulonephritis, oral ulceration, glossitis, and nightmares

Main signs & symptoms: Vexatious heat in the heart and chest, thirst, red face, thirst with a desire for chilled drinks, reddish, astringent, inhibited urination, possible oral and tongue ulceration, a red tongue, and rapid pulse

Contraindications:

1. Do not use in case of diarrhea.

Formula explanation:

Raw Rehmannia cools the blood and enriches yin, thus restraining heart fire. Akebia clears heat from the heart channel above, while below, it also clears heat from the small intestine. In addition, it disinhibits water and opens strangury. Raw Licorice clears heat and resolves toxins and regulates and harmonizes the other medicinals. In particular, it is believed that using Licorice's small root tips stops strangury and pain. Bamboo Leaves clear the heart and eliminate vexation.

Additions & subtractions:

For severe oral ulceration and sores on the tongue, add Rhizoma Coptidis Chinensis (*Huang Lian*).

Also, one can add *Wu Ling San* (Five *Ling* Powder), *i.e.*, Rhizoma Alismatis (*Ze Xie*), Sclerotium Poriae Cocos (*Fu Ling*), Sclerotium Polypori Umbellati (*Zhu Ling*), Rhizoma Atractylodis Macrocephalae (*Bai Zhu*), and Ramulus Cinnamomi (*Gui Zhi*).

For hematuria, subtract Bamboo Leaves add Herba Cephalanoplos (*Xiao Ji*) and Herba Ecliptae Prostratae (*Han Lian Cao*) or add Cephalanoplos and Rhizoma Imperatae Cylindricae (*Bai Mao Gen*).

For severe urinary tract infection, add Herba Cephalanoplos (*Xiao Ji*), Fructus Gardeniae Jasminoidis (*Zhi Zi*), and Semen Plantaginis (*Che Qian Zi*).

For concomitant or more severe yin vacuity, add Herba Dendrobii (*Shi Hu*) and Rhizoma Anemarrhenae (*Zhi Mu*).

B. *Long Dan Xie Gan Tang* (Gentiana Scabra Drain the Liver Decoction)

Composition:

Radix Gentianae Scabrae (*Long Dan Cao*), 6g, stir-fried in wine
Radix Scutellariae Baicalensis (*Huang Qin*), 9g
Fructus Gardeniae Jasminoidis (*Shan Zhi Zi*), 9g, stir-fried in wine
Rhizoma Alismatis (*Ze Xie*), 12g
Caulis Akebiae Mutong (*Mu Tong*), 9g
Semen Plantaginis (*Che Qian Zi*), 9g
Radix Angelicae Sinensis (*Dang Gui*), 3g, washed in wine
raw Radix Rehmanniae (*Sheng Di*), 9g, stir-fried in wine
Radix Bupleuri (*Chai Hu*), 6g
raw Radix Glycyrrhizae (*Sheng Gan Cao*), 6g

Functions: Drains liver/gallbladder replete heat, clears lower burner damp heat

Indications: 1) Liver/gallbladder replete heat harassing above or 2) damp heat pouring below. Acute conjunctivitis, uveitis, corneal ulcers, acute glaucoma, central retinitis, acute otitis media, boils and carbuncles in the vestibular and external auditory canal, nasal furuncles, hypertension, acute icteric hepatitis, acute cholecystitis, herpes zoster, herpes genitalia, cold sores, acute pyelonephritis, acute cystitis, urethritis, acute pelvic inflammation, acute prostatitis, orchitis, epididymitis, vaginitis, abnormal vaginal discharge, vaginal itching, lymphadenitis of the groin, hyperthyroidism, migraine headache, eczema in general and scrotal eczema in particular, and intercostal neuralgia

Main signs & symptoms: 1) Headache, red eyes, lateral costal pian, a bitter taste in the mouth, loss of hearing, swelling of the ears; 2) Genital swelling, genital itching, impotence, genital sweating, urinary strangury, turbid urine, damp heat abnormal vaginal discharge in women, a red tongue with yellow coating, and a rapid, forceful pulse

Contraindications:

1. Do not use in large doses or for prolonged periods of time in patients with spleen/stomach vacuity.
2. Do not use in large doses or for prolonged periods of time in patients with damaged body fluids.
3. Do not use in cases with a red tongue but scanty coating.

Formula explanation:

Within this formula, Gentiana Scabra, greatly bitter and greatly cold, is the sovereign for both draining fire and eliminating dampness. It drains replete liver/gallbladder fire from the upper (body). It also precipitates and clears damp heat from the lower (body). Scutellaria and Gardenia are the ministers. They also have the functions of draining fire with bitterness and cold and are combined with Gentian Scabra for that purpose. Alisma, Akebia, and Plantaginis clear heat and disinhibit dampness. They, therefore, assist in eliminating damp heat via the urinary tract. Because the liver stores the blood and heat within the liver channel can easily damage yin and blood, at the same

75

time as using bitter cold ingredients to dry dampness, raw **Rehmannia** and *Dang Gui* are used as assistants to enrich yin and nourish the blood. Licorice regulates and harmonizes all the other medicinals. Therefore, within this formula there is supplementation within drainage and enrichment within disinhibition. This assists the downbearing of fire and the clearing of heat and the separation of clear from damp turbidity.

Additions & subtractions:

In case of acute icteric hepatitis, subtract Alisma and Plantago and add Herba Artemisiae Capillaris (*Yin Chen*).

Also for jaundice, subtract Licorice and add Herba Artemisiae Capillaris (*Yin Chen*) and Radix Et Rhizoma Rhei (*Da Huang*).

For a reddish vaginal discharge and a wiry, rapid pulse, add Radix Rubrus Paeoniae Lactiflorae (*Chi Shao*) and Stamen Nelumbinis Nuciferae (*Lian Xu*).

For yellow or red and white abnormal vaginal discharge with foul odor, subtract Licorice and Scutellaria and add Cortex Phellodendri (*Huang Bai*).

For severe headache and red, painful eyes, add Flos Chrysanthemi Morifolii (*Ju Hua*) and Folium Mori Albi (*Sang Ye*).

For hemoptysis due to liver fire damaging the lungs, add Cortex Radicis Moutan (*Dan Pi*) and Cacumen Biotae Orientalis (*Ce Bai Ye*).

For spasms and convulsions, add Ramulus Uncariae Cum Uncis (*Gou Teng*) and Bulbus Fritillariae Cirrhosae (*Chuan Bei Mu*).

Comment: This formula can also be used effectively in combination with Western antibiotics.

C. *Bai Tou Weng Tang* (Pulsatilla Decoction)

Composition:

Radix Pulsatillae Chinensis (*Bai Tou Weng*), 15g
Cortex Phellodendri (*Huang Bai*), 12g
Rhizoma Coptidis Chinensis (*Huang Lian*), 6g
Cortex Fraxini (*Qin Pi*), 12g

Functions: Clears heat and resolves toxins, cools the blood and stops dysentery

Indications: Hot dysentery. Acute enteritis, postpartum enteritis, acute bacillary dysentery, amebic dysentery, ulcerative colitis, abnormal vaginal discharge, urinary tract infection, and acute conjunctivitis

Main signs & symptoms: Diarrhea with abdominal pain, tenesmus, burning heat around the anus, diarrhea containing pus and blood with more red colored material and less white colored material, thirst with a desire to drink chilled water, a red tongue with yellow coating, and a wiry, rapid pulse

Contraindications:

1. Do not use in patients with spleen vacuity.
2. Do not use long-term.

Formula explanation:

Pulsatilla is the main medicinal in this formula for clearing heat toxins from the blood division. Coptis, bitter and cold, clears damp heat and especially from the intestines and stomach. Phellodendron drains damp heat from the lower burner. Together these two are the assistant medicinals for clearing and resolving and cooling the blood. Fraxinus' nature is cold and its flavor is bitter and astringent. It has the functions of restraining, astringing, and stopping dysentery. When combined together with the above medicinals, the entire formula thus clears heat and resolves toxins, cools the blood and stops dysentery.

Additions & subtractions:

For colitis with predominance of heat, add from the following: Flos Lonicerae Japonicae (*Yin Hua*), Radix Rubrus Paeoniae Lactiflorae (*Chi Shao*), Caulis Sargentodoxae (*Hong Teng*), Herba Patriniae Heterophyllae (*Bai Jiang Cao*), and Herba Kummerowiae Striatae (*Ma Yi Cao*).

For colitis with predominance of dampness, add from the following: Rhizoma Atractylodis (*Cang Zhu*), Cortex Magnoliae Officinalis (*Hou Po*), Semen Coicis Lachryma-jobi (*Yi Yi Ren*), and Semen Plantaginis (*Che Qian Zi*).

For colitis with food stagnation, add from the following: Semen Arecae Catechu (*Bing Lang*), Fructus Immaturus Citri Seu Ponciri (*Zhi Shi*), Fructus Crataegi (*Shan Zha*), and Massa Medica Fermentata (*Shen Qu*).

For severe abdominal pain and tenesmus, add Radix Saussureae Seu Vladimiriae (*Mu Xiang*), Fructus Citri Seu Ponciri (*Zhi Ke*), Radix Albus Paeoniae Lactiflorae (*Bai Shao*), and Radix Angelicae Sinensis (*Dang Gui*).

Also for severe abdominal pain, add Radix Saussureae Seu Vladimiriae (*Mu Xiang*) and Semen Arecae Catechu (*Bing Lang*).

For concurrent signs of an exterior patterns, such as fever and aversion to cold, add Radix Puerariae Lobatae (*Ge Gen*), Radix Scutellariae Baicalensis (*Huang Qin*), Flos Lonicerae Japonicae (*Yin Hua*), and Fructus Forsythiae Suspensae (*Lian Qiao*).

78

For severe heat and more obvious heat toxins, add Herba Portulacae Oleraceae (*Ma Chi Xian*) and Flos Lonicerae Japonicae (*Yin Hua*).

For concomitant blood vacuity, for instance postpartum, add Gelatinum Corii Asini (*E Jiao*) and Radix Glycyrrhizae (*Gan Cao*). This results in *Bai Tou Weng Jia Gan Cao E Jiao Tang* (Pulsatilla, Licorice, & Donkey Skin Glue Decoction).

For red and white dysentery, add Cortex Radicis Moutan (*Dan Pi*) and raw Radix Rehmanniae (*Sheng Di*).

If there is urinary frequency, urgency, and pain, add Caulis Akebiae Mutong (*Mu Tong*), Rhizoma Imperatae Cylindricae (*Bai Mao Gen*), and Herba Desmodii (*Jin Qian Cao*).

For red, swollen, painful eyes, add Flos Chrysanthemi Morifolii (*Ju Hua*), Cortex Radicis Moutan (*Dan Pi*), and Flos Carthami Tinctorii (*Hong Hua*).

For amebic dysentery, add Pericarpium Punicae Granati (*Shi Liu Pi*).

For bacillary dysentery, add Radix Sanguisorbae (*Di Yu*), Herba Agrimoniae Pilosae (*Xian He Cao*), and Radix Saussureae Seu Vladimiriae (*Mu Xiang*).

For coma and convulsions due to extreme fluid loss in turn due to dysentery, add *An Gong Niu Huang Wan* (Quiet the Palace Bezoar Pills) or *Zi Xue Dan* (Purple Snow Elixir).

For dryness in the upper burner due to damp heat below, add Radix Glehniae Littoralis (*Sha Shen*) and Tuber Ophiopogonis Japonicae (*Mai Dong*).

Comment: This formula is very effective for both amebic and bacillary dysentery. Travellers to countries where dysentery is prevalent should carry a supply with them. If amebic dysentery is left untreated, the amoebae may invade the liver, resulting in amoebic hepatitis. The stools associated with amebic dysentery look like chocolate pudding.

4.6 *Qing Xu Re Ji* (Formulas for clearing vacuity heat)

Representative formula: *Qing Hao Bie Jia Tang* (Artemisia Apiacea & Carapax Amydae Decoction)

Composition:

Herba Artemisiae Apiaceae (*Qing Hao*), 6g
Carapax Amydae (*Bie Jia*), 15g
raw Radix Rehmanniae (*Xi Sheng Di*), 12g
Rhizoma Anemarrhenae (*Zhi Mu*), 6g
Cortex Radicis Moutan (*Dan Pi*), 9g

Functions: Nourishes yin, penetrates heat

Indications: Latter stages of warm diseases, yin fluids consumed and damaged, evils hidden in the yin division. Advanced stages of various infectious diseases, pulmonary tuberculosis, chronic nephritis, kidney tuberculosis, fevers of unknown etiology, typhoid fever convalescence, and post-surgical fevers

Main signs & symptoms: Evening heat, morning coolness, absence of sweating as fever recedes, emaciation with no loss of appetite, a red tongue with scant coating, and a fine, rapid pulse

Contraindications:

1. Do not use during the early stage of a warm disease.
2. Do not use with spasms and convulsions.

Formula explanation:

In this formula, Carapax Amydae enriches yin and recedes fever. It enters the network vessels and tracks down evils. Artemisia Apiacea, sweet-smelling and fragrant, clears heat and penetrates (*i.e.*, vents) the network vessels. It leads evils to be discharged to the outside. Raw Rehmannia is sweet and cool and enriches yin. Anemarrhena is bitter and cold and enriches and moistens. When combined with Carapax Amydae, these three have the function of nourishing yin and penetrating heat. Moutan combined with Artemisia Apiacea clears heat hidden within the blood on the inside and penetrates hidden yin evils on the outside.

Additions & subtractions:

For severe yin vacuity, add Tuber Ophiopogonis Japonicae (*Mai Dong*), Radix Albus Paeoniae Lactiflorae (*Bai Shao*), and Radix Scrophulariae Ningpoensis (*Xuan Shen*).

For severe heat, add Radix Stellariae (*Yin Chai Hu*), Herba Ecliptae Prostratae (*Han Lian Cao*), and Radix Cynanchi Baiwei (*Bai Wei*).

For blazing fire due to vacuity or fevers due to unknown etiology with yin vacuity, add Radix Cynanchi Baiwei (*Bai Wei*) and Cortex Radicis Lycii (*Di Gu Pi*).

For pulmonary tuberculosis, add Radix Glehniae Littoralis (*Sha Shen*) and Herba Ecliptae Prostratae (*Han Lian Cao*).

For pulmonary tuberculosis with chest fullness and oppression, add Pericarpium Trichosanthis Kirlowii (*Gua Lou Pi*).

For pediatric summertime night fevers but morning coolness, add Radix Cynanchi Baiwei (*Bai Wei*) and Ramulus Nelumbinis Nuciferae (*Lian Geng*).

For kidney tuberculosis or pyelonephritis with heat in the palms of the hands, soles of the feet, and heart with yellow urine and a red tongue with yellow coating, add Rhizoma Imperatae Cylindricae (*Bai Mao Gen*).

5

Wen Li Ji
Warming the Interior Formulas

The formulas in this chapter are composed mainly of warm and hot medicinals. Interior cold may be due to either external invasion of cold having reached the interior or from internal generation of cold due to yang vacuity. In addition, improper use of cool and cold medicinals may result in damage to the yang qi, as can overeating raw and cold foods and drinking chilled liquids. Within this chapter there are three subcategories of formulas. These are 1) formulas which warm the center and dispel cold, 2) formulas which secure yang and save counterflow, and 3) formulas which warm the channels and scatter cold. For relatively superficial conditions, formulas which warm the channels and scatter cold are used. For cold affecting the middle burner, formulas which warm the center and dispel cold are used. For extreme conditions associated with cold which has devastated yang, formulas which secure yang and save counterflow are used.

Cautions & Contraindications:

1. These formulas must be used with care in patients with yin vacuity or blood loss.
2. Do not use these formulas with true heat/false cold.
3. The dosage of the hot, drying medicinals in these formulas must be adjusted based on the season, climate, and the bodily constitution of the patient.

5.1 *Wen Zhong Qu Han Ji* (Formulas for warming the center & dispelling cold)

Representative formula: *Li Zhong Wan* (Rectify the Center Pills)

Composition:

Radix Panacis Ginseng (*Ren Shen*), 6g
dry Rhizoma Zingiberis (*Gan Jiang*), 5g
Radix Glycyrrhizae (*Gan Cao*), 6g, mix-fried
Rhizoma Atractylodis Macrocephalae (*Bai Zhu*), 9g

Functions: Warms the center and dispels cold, supplements the qi and fortifies the spleen

Indications: 1) Middle burner vacuity cold, 2) yang vacuity, loss of blood, and 3) pediatric chronic fright (*i.e.*, convulsions). Acute and chronic gastritis, gastric or duodenal ulcers, gastroptosis, gastrectasis, irritable bowel syndrome, chronic colitis, cholera-like disorders, chronic bronchitis, oral herpes, functional uterine bleeding, bloody stools due to gastroduodenal ulcer, angina pectoris, and anemia

Main signs & symptoms: Diarrhea but no thirst, nausea and vomiting, abdominal pain, no desire for food or drinks, possible cholera-like conditions, a pale tongue with a white coating, and a deep, fine pulse

Contraindications:

1. Do not use for externally contracted diseases with fever even though accompanied by chills.
2. Do not use in cases with yin vacuity.

3. When used with cholera-like conditions, discontinue use after vomiting and diarrhea have stopped.

Formula explanation:

Within this formula, acrid, hot, dry Ginger is the sovereign. It warms the middle burner spleen and stomach and dispels interior cold. Ginseng greatly supplements the source qi. It assists transportation and transformation and rectifies upbearing and downbearing. It is the minister medicinal. Atractylodis fortifies the spleen and dries dampness. Mix-fried Licorice boosts the qi and harmonizes the center. It is used as both assistant and messenger. When these four medicinals are combined, cold in the middle burner obtains acrid heat and is eliminated, while middle burner vacuity obtains sweet warmth and is augmented. Thus the clear yang is upborne and the turbid yin is downborne, transportation and transformation are fortified and the middle burner is cured.

Additions & subtractions:

For severe vomiting, subtract Atractylodis and add raw Rhizoma Zingiberis (*Sheng Jiang*) and Flos Caryophylli (*Ding Xiang*).

Also for vomiting, add Flos Caryophylli (*Ding Xiang*) and Fructus Evodiae Rutecarpae (*Wu Zhu Yu*). This results in *Ding Yu Li Zhong Tang* (Clove & Evodia Rectify the Center Decoction).

For vomiting of watery substance and coughing with copious thin, white phlegm, add Rhizoma Pinelliae Ternatae (*Ban Xia*) and Sclerotium Poriae Cocos (*Fu Ling*). This results in *Li Zhong Hua Tan Wan* (Rectify the Center, Transform Phlegm Pills).

For pain due to roundworms, subtract Licorice and add Pericarpium Zanthoxyli Bungeani (*Chuan Jiao*), Fructus Pruni Mume (*Wu Mei*), and Sclerotium Poriae Cocos (*Fu Ling*). This results in *Li Zhong An Hui Wan* (Rectify the Center, Quiet Roundworms Pills).

For vomiting of sour fluid, add Rhizoma Coptidis Chinensis (*Huang Lian*). This results in *Lian Li Tang* (Coptis Rectifying Decoction).

For more prominent cold, add Radix Praeparatus Aconiti Carmichaeli (*Fu Zi*). This results in *Fu Zi Li Zhong Wan* (Aconite Rectify the Center Pills).

For dual spleen/kidney yang vacuity, add Cortex Cinnamomi (*Rou Gui*) and Radix Praeparatus Aconiti Carmichaeli (*Fu Zi*). This results in *Gui Fu Li Zhong Tang* (Cinnamon & Aconite Rectify the Center Decoction).

For glomus and abdominal distention and fullness due to vacuity cold of the spleen, add Fructus Immaturus Citri Seu Ponciri (*Zhi Shi*) and Sclerotium Poria Cocos (*Fu Ling*). This results in *Zhi Shi Li Zhong Wan* (Immature Citrus Rectify the Center Pills).

For severe diarrhea, add Radix Dioscoreae Oppositae (*Shan Yao*), Semen Dolichos Lablabis (*Bian Dou*), and Sclerotium Poriae Cocos (*Fu Ling*).

For loss of blood due to yang vacuity, add Gelatinum Corii Asini (*E Jiao*), Folium Artemisiae Argyii (*Ai Ye*), and Gelatinum Cornu Cervi (*Lu Jiao Jiao*).

Also for bleeding due to yang vacuity, replace dry Ginger with blast-fried Rhizoma Zingiberis (*Pao Jiang*) and add Radix Astragali Membranacei (*Huang Qi*), Radix Angelicae Sinensis (*Dang Gui*), and Gelatinum Corii Asini (*E Jiao*).

If there is pain in the chest, add Radix Salviae Miltiorrhizae (*Dan Shen*), Fructus Trichosanthis Kirlowii (*Gua Lou*), Tuber Curcumae (*Yu Jin*), and Fructus Citri Seu Ponciri (*Zhi Ke*).

For infantile convulsions, add Ramulus Uncariae Cum Uncis (*Gou Teng*), Rhizoma Gastrodiae Elatae (*Tian Ma*), and Bombyx Batryticatus (*Jiang Can*).

For abnormal vaginal discharge due to downward pouring to dampness due to vacuity cold of the spleen, add Semen Cuscutae (*Tu Si Zi*), Cornu Degelatinum Cervi (*Lu Jiao Shuang*), Radix Dioscoreae Oppositae (*Shan Yao*), Sclerotium Poriae Cocos (*Fu Ling*), stir-fried Semen Coicis Lachryma-jobi (*Chao Yi Ren*), and Concha Ostreae (*Mu Li*).

For palpitations, add Sclerotium Poriae Cocos (*Fu Ling*).

For more prominent abdominal pain, add Radix Saussureae Seu Vladimiriae (*Mu Xiang*).

For stagnation of qi, add Pericarpium Citri Reticulatae (*Chen Pi*) or Fructus Citri Sacrodactylis (*Fo Shou*).

For edema, add Sclerotium Poriae Cocos (*Fu Ling*), Rhizoma Alismatis (*Ze Xie*), and Cortex Benincasae Hispidae (*Dong Gua Pi*).

For chronic diarrhea which will not stop, add Semen Myristicae Fragrantis (*Rou Dou Kou*), Semen Dolichos Lablabis (*Bai Bian Dou*), Radix Dioscoreae Oppositae (*Shan Yao*), and Fructus Terminaliae Chebulae (*He Zi*).

5.2 *Hui Yang Jiu Ni Ji* (Formulas for returning the yang & stemming counterflow)

Representative formula: *Si Ni Tang* (Four Counterflows Decoction)

Composition:

raw Radix Aconiti Carmichaeli (*Sheng Fu Zi*), 5-10g
dry Rhizoma Zingiberis (*Gan Jiang*), 9g
Radix Glycyrrhizae (*Gan Cao*), 6g, mix-fried

Functions: Returns yang and stems counterflow

Indications: 1) *Shao yin* diseases, 2) collapse of yang due to erroneously sweating *tai yang* diseases. Influenza, intestinal fever, cholera, diarrhea, neurotic vomiting, indigestion, edema, jaundice, hypopituitarism, hypothyroidism, adrenal insufficiency, intractable arthritis, prostration, heart failure, cardiac insufficiency, and coma

Main signs & symptoms: Inversion counterflow of the four extremities, aversion to cold, sleeping with knees drawn up, nausea and vomiting, no thirst, abdominal pain, diarrhea, fatigued spirit, desire to sleep (all the time), a white, glossy tongue coating, and a minute, fine pulse

Contraindications:

1. Do not use in cases of true heat/false cold.

Formula explanation:

In this formula, Aconite, greatly acrid and greatly hot, is the sovereign. It is pure yang but does have toxins. It supplements and boosts the former heaven (*i.e.*, prenatal) fire of the gate of life. It opens and moves the 12 channels. Used raw, it is able to warm yang and dispel cold. Dry Ginger warms middle burner yang and eliminates interior cold. It assists Aconite in stretching and emitting yang qi and is the minister medicinal. As mentioned above, raw Aconite has large toxins and dry Ginger is harsh in nature. Licorice is the assistant medicinal which boosts the qi and warms the center. It is also able to resolve toxins and thus reduces Aconite's toxicity and Ginger's drying properties.

Additions & subtractions:

For chronic rheumatoid arthritis due to cold *bi*, add Ramulus Cinnamomi (*Gui Zhi*) and Radix Albus Paeoniae Lactiflorae (*Bai Shao*).

For edema or abnormal vaginal discharge due to cold from spleen/kidney dual vacuity, add Radix Codonopsis Pilosulae (*Dang Shen*), Sclerotium Poriae Cocos (*Fu Ling*), and Rhizoma Alismatis (*Ze Xie*).

If diarrhea stops suddenly but the limbs remain cold, add Radix Panacis Ginseng (*Ren Shen*). This results in *Si Ni Jia Ren Shen Tang* (Four Counterflows Plus Ginseng Decoction).

Comment: Today Radix Praeparatus Aconiti Carmichaeli (*Shu Fu Zi*) is almost always used instead of raw Aconite. However, in serious cases such as interior cold with exterior heat, raw Aconite should be used since it is stronger. In that case, decoct it separately for 30 minutes—1 hour before adding the other medicinals.

5.3 *Wen Jing San Han Ji* (Formulas for warming the channels and scattering cold)

Representative formula: *Dang Gui Si Ni Tang* (*Dang Gui* Four Counterflows Decoction)

Composition:

Radix Angelicae Sinensis (*Dang Gui*), 12g
Ramulus Cinnamomi (*Gui Zhi*), 9g, remove the skin
Radix Paeoniae Lactiflorae (*Shao Yao*), 9g
Herba Cum Radice Asari (*Xi Xin*), 1.5g
Radix Glycyrrhizae (*Gan Cao*), 5g, mix-fried
Caulis Akebiae Mutong (*Mu Tong*), 3g
Fructus Zizyphi Jujubae (*Da Zao*), 8 pieces

Functions: Warms the channels and scatters cold, nourishes blood and opens the vessels

Indications: 1) Yang qi insufficiency with concomitant blood vacuity, external invasion of cold evils, 2) cold entering the channels and network vessels. Thromboangiitis obliterans, varicose veins, frostbite (before skins swells and cracks or after healed), callouses and corns, dysmenorrhea, hernia, colic testalgia, chronic rheumatoid arthritis, Raynaud's disease, fibromyalgia, sciatica, peptic ulcer, chronic urticaria, midline pain, chilblains, and gangrene

Main signs & symptoms: Inversion cold of the hands and feet, a pale tongue with white coating, and a deep, fine pulse or a fine, weak, almost imperceptible pulse

Contraindications:

1. Use cautiously during the spring and summer or in warm climates.

2. Do not use in patients with fire due to yin vacuity.

Formula explanation:

Within this formula, *Dang Gui* is bitter, acrid, sweet, and warm. It supplements and harmonizes the blood. Combined with Peony, these two supplement blood vacuity and are the sovereign medicinals in this formula. Cinnamon is acrid, sweet, and warm. It warms the channels and scatters cold. Combined with Asarum, these two scatter cold from both the inside and outside. They are the minister medicinals in this formula. Licorice and Red Dates are sweet. They boost the qi and fortify the spleen. In addition, they help *Dang Gui* and Peony supplement the blood and Asarum and Cinnamon open yang. Licorice and Red Dates are the assistant medicinals. Further, Akebia opens the channels and vessels. It is the messenger medicinal in this formula. Once blood vacuity is remedied and yang qi is restored, the hands and feet become warm automatically.

Additions & subtractions:

For dysmenorrhea and *shan*, add Radix Linderae Strychnifoliae (*Wu Yao*), Fructus Foeniculi Vulgaris (*Xiao Hui Xiang*), and Rhizoma Alpiniae Officinari (*Gao Liang Jiang*).

For dysmenorrhea due to blood vacuity with cold evils, subtract Akebia and add prepared Radix Rehmanniae (*Shu Di*) to nourish the blood and regulate menstruation.

Also for cold pain in the lower abdomen with menstruation, add Herba Leonuri Heterophylli (*Yi Mu Cao*) and Rhizoma Cyperi Rotundi (*Xiang Fu*).

For persistent, mild headache, vertigo, and ringing in the ears, add Radix Angelicae (*Bai Zhi*) and Radix Ledebouriellae Sesloidis (*Fang Feng*).

For vague upper abdominal pain which gets better with warmth or pressure and vomiting of clear fluids, add Fructus Evodiae Rutecarpae (*Wu Zhu Yu*), Fructus Citri Sacrodactylis (*Fo Shou*), and Radix Codonopsis Pilosulae (*Dang Shen*).

For chronic sciatica which will not heal, add Radix Praeparatus Aconiti Carmichaeli (*Fu Zi*), Radix Et Rhizoma Rhei (*Da Huang*), Radix Dipsaci (*Xu Duan*), and Rhizoma Cibotii Barometsis (*Gou Ji*).

For loose stools, nausea, and vomiting, add raw Rhizoma Zingiberis (*Sheng Jiang*) and Fructus Evodiae Rutecarpae (*Wu Zhu Yu*). This results in *Dang Gui Si Ni Jia Wu Zhu Yu Sheng Jiang Tang* (*Dang Gui* Four Counterflows Plus Evodia & Fresh Ginger Decoction).

For cold colic testalgia, add Fructus Foeniculi Vulgaris (*Xiao Hui Xiang*) to warm the liver and rectify the qi.

6

Bu Yi Ji
Supplementing & Boosting Formulas

Formulas which enrich and nourish and supplement and boost insufficiency of the body's qi and blood and yin and yang are called supplementing formulas. This category of formulas is further divided into 4 subcategories: 1) formulas which supplement the qi, 2) formulas which supplement the blood, 3) formulas which supplement yin, and 4) formulas which supplement yang. Because of the interrelationship between the qi and blood and between yin and yang, frequently formulas which supplement the qi will contain medicinals which nourish blood and *vice versa*. Likewise, formulas which supplement yin will often contain ingredients to strengthen yang and *vice versa*. Nevertheless, when using supplementing formulas, the practitioner must accurately identify whether qi, blood, yin, or yang is predominantly vacuous and should choose a formula from the appropriate category. Because Chinese medicine works by restoring balance to the system, supplementing formulas should not be used unless there is diagnosable vacuity and insufficiency.

Methods of Preparation & Administration:

Supplementing formulas are usually cooked over a low heat for a prolonged period of time. If Ginseng is used, it is commonly decocted in a special double boiler and this decoction is added to the other decocted medicinals. Supplementing formulas are best taken on an empty stomach.

6.1 *Bu Qi Ji* (Qi-supplementing formulas)

Representative formulas:

A. *Si Jun Zi Tang* (Four Gentlemen Decoction)

Composition:

Radix Panacis Ginseng (*Ren Shen*), 10g
Rhizoma Atractylodis Macrocephalae (*Bai Zhu*), 9g
Sclerotium Poriae Cocos (*Fu Ling*), 9g
Radix Glycyrrhizae (*Gan Cao*), 6g, mix-fried

Functions: Boosts the qi and fortifies the spleen

Indications: Spleen and stomach qi vacuity. Chronic gastritis, gastric and duodenal ulcer, gastrointestinal weakness and dysfunction, gastroptosis, irritable bowel syndrome, diabetes mellitus, periodic paralysis, uterine fibroids, anemia, vomiting, and diarrhea

Main signs & symptoms: A faded, white facial color, a faint, lethargic voice, diminished appetite, lack of strength of the four extremities, loose stools, a pale tongue, and a fine, relaxed/retarded pulse

Contraindications:

1. Do not use without modification in high fever, yin vacuity with exuberant fire, accumulation and stagnation with qi distention, or fluid insufficiency.
2. Prolonged use may result in a dry mouth, vexatious thirst, agitation, easy anger, and constipation.

Formula explanation:

Ginseng is the sovereign medicinal in this formula. It is sweet and warm and greatly supplements the source qi. It also fortifies the spleen and nourishes the stomach. Atractylodis is the minister. It is bitter and warm and fortifies the spleen and dries dampness. The assistant is Poria which is sweet and bland and percolates dampness and fortifies the spleen. Used together, Poria and Atractylodis' ability to fortify the spleen and eliminate dampness are strengthened, thus promoting transportation and transformation. The messenger is mix-fried Licorice. It is sweet and warm and regulates the center. Taken as a whole, this formula has the functions of boosting the qi and fortifying the spleen.

Additions & subtractions:

For qi stagnation manifest by chest oppression and fullness, add Pericarpium Citri Reticulatae (*Ju Pi*). This results in *Wu Wei Yi Gong San* (Five Flavors Extraordinary Merit Powder).

For cough with copious, white, thin phlegm or for more prominent dampness, add Pericarpium Citri Reticulatae (*Chen Pi*), Rhizoma Pinelliae Ternatae (*Ban Xia*), raw Rhizoma Zingiberis (*Sheng Jiang*), and Fructus Zizyphi Jujubae (*Da Zao*). This results in *Liu Jun Zi Tang* (Six Gentlemen Decoction).

For distention and fullness in the epigastrium, vomiting, diarrhea, and abdominal pain, to *Liu Jun Zi Tang* add Radix Saussureae Seu Vladimiriae (*Mu Xiang*) and Fructus Amomi (*Sha Ren*). This results in *Xiang Sha Liu Jun Zi Tang* (Amomum & Saussurea Six Gentlemen Decoction).

For qi and blood vacuity, add *Si Wu Tang* (Four Materials Decoction). This results in *Ba Zhen Tang* (Eight Pearls Decoction).

For more serious qi and blood vacuity with cold limbs, add *Si Wu Tang* plus Cortex Cinnamomi (*Rou Gui*) and Radix Astragali Membranacei (*Huang Qi*). This results in *Shi Quan Da Bu Tang* (Ten Complete Great Supplementing Decoction).

For weakness of the spleen and dampness with vomiting, diarrhea, and poor appetite, add Radix Astragali Membranacei (*Huang Qi*) and Semen Dolichos Lablabis (*Bai Bian Dou*).

For acute gastric disorder and ulcer, to *Liu Jun Zi Tang* add Radix Scutellariae Baicalensis (*Huang Qin*), Rhizoma Coptidis Chinensis (*Huang Lian*), and Concha Ostreae (*Mu Li*). This results in *Ban Xie Liu Jun Zi Tang* (Pinellia Draining Six Gentlemen Decoction).

For chronic gastric disorder and ulcer or pediatric spleen vacuity disorders, add Semen Dolichos Lablabis (*Bian Dou*), Radix Dioscoreae Oppositae (*Shan Yao*), Fructus Cardamomi (*Bai Dou Kou*), Semen Nelumbinis Nuciferae (*Lian Zi*), Radix Platycodi Grandiflori (*Jie Geng*), and Semen Coicis Lachryma-jobi (*Yi Ren*). This results in *Shen Ling Bai Zhu San* (Ginseng, Poria, & Atractylodis Powder).

For chronic gastrointestinal complaints with pain, to *Xiang Sha Liu Jun Zi Tang* add Cortex Magnoliae Officinalis (*Hou Po*) and Rhizoma Cyperi Rotundi (*Xiang Fu*). This results in *Xiang Sha Yang Wei Tang* (Saussurea & Amomum Nourish the Stomach Decoction).

For indigestion, loss of appetite, and diarrhea due to food stagnation, add Semen Nelumbinis Nuciferae (*Lian Zi*), Radix Dioscoreae Oppositae (*Shan Yao*), Fructus Crataegi (*Shan Zha*), Pericarpium Citri Reticulatae (*Chen Pi*), and Rhizoma Alismatis (*Ze Xie*). This results in *Fen Xiao Tang* (Dividing & Dispersing Decoction).

For summerheat pattern with diarrhea, add Radix Puerariae Lobatae (*Ge Gen*), Herba Agastachis Seu Pogostemi (*Huo Xiang*), and Radix

Saussureae Seu Vladimiriae (*Mu Xiang*). This results in *Qian Shi Bai Zhu San* (Master Qian's Atractylodis Powder).

For recent onset edema with scanty, yellow urine, poor appetite, edema worse in the morning, and fatigue, add Herba Eupatorii (*Pei Lan*), Herba Agastachis Seu Pogostemi (*Huo Xiang*), Caulis Akebiae Mutong (*Mu Tong*), and Semen Coicis Lachryma-jobi (*Yi Ren*).

For edema of the limbs with a sensation of bodily heaviness and lassitude, add Semen Plantaginis (*Che Qian Zi*), Herba Ephedrae (*Ma Huang*), Rhizoma Atractylodis (*Cang Zhu*), Radix Angelicae Pubescentis (*Du Huo*), and Ramus Loranthi Seu Visci (*Ji Sheng*).

If edema is accompanied by chest oppression, dyspnea, copious phlegm, and scanty urine, add *Wu Ling San* (Five *Ling* Powder), *i.e.*, Rhizoma Alismatis (*Ze Xie*), Sclerotium Poriae Cocos (*Fu Ling*), Sclerotium Polypori Umbellati (*Zhu Ling*), Rhizoma Atractylodis Macrocephalae (*Bai Zhu*), and Ramulus Cinnamomi (*Gui Zhi*).

For nausea and vomiting during pregnancy, add Fructus Amomi (*Sha Ren*), Pericarpium Citri Reticulatae (*Chen Pi*), Rhizoma Pinelliae Ternatae (*Ban Xia*), and Cortex Magnoliae Officinalis (*Hou Po*).

For edema during pregnancy, add *Wu Pi Tin* (Five Peels Drink), *i.e.*, Cortex Sclerotii Poriae Cocos (*Fu Ling Pi*), Cortex Radicis Mori (*Sang Bai Pi*), raw Cortex Rhizomatis Zingiberis (*Sheng Jiang Pi*), Pericarpium Arecae Catechu (*Da Fu Pi*), and Pericarpium Citri Reticulatae (*Chen Pi*).

For menstrual pain due to qi and blood vacuity, add Rhizoma Ligustici Wallichii (*Chuan Xiong*), Radix Salviae Miltiorrhizae (*Dan Shen*), Rhizoma Corydalis Yanhusuo (*Yan Hu*), Caulis Millettiae Seu Spatholobi (*Ji Xue Teng*), and Herba Leonuri Heterophylli (*Yi Mu Cao*).

For post-menstrual pain, add Radix Angelicae Sinensis (*Dang Gui*), Radix Albus Paeoniae Lactiflorae (*Bai Shao*), Fructus Zizyphi Jujubae (*Da Zao*), Folium Artemisiae Argyii (*Ai Ye*), and Semen Cuscutae (*Tu Si Zi*).

For postpartum dizziness and vertigo, to *Ba Zhen Tang* add Radix Angelicae (*Bai Zhi*) and Ramulus Uncariae Cum Uncis (*Gou Teng*) or add Radix Astragali Membranacei (*Huang Qi*), raw Rhizoma Zingiberis (*Sheng Jiang*), and Fructus Zizyphi Jujubae (*Da Zao*).

For abnormal vaginal discharge due to damp turbidity pouring downward, add Radix Astragali Membranacei (*Huang Qi*), Radix Angelicae Sinensis (*Dang Gui*), Fructus Immaturus Citri Seu Ponciri (*Zhi Shi*), and Herba Dianthi (*Qu Mai*).

For slightly yellowish vaginal discharge accompanied by fullness and oppression of the chest, heaviness of the lower extremities, and a thick, white, slimy tongue coating, replace Poria with Cortex Sclerotii Poriae Cocos (*Fu Ling Pi*) and mix-fried Licorice with raw Radix Glycyrrhizae (*Sheng Gan Cao*) and add Rhizoma Atractylodis (*Cang Zhu*), Cortex Phellodendri (*Huang Bai*), Cortex Radicis Moutan (*Dan Pi*), Herba Artemisiae Anomalae (*Liu Ji Nu*), and Rhizoma Drynariae (*Gu Sui Bu*).

Comment: Do not substitute Radix Codonopsis Pilosulae (*Dang Shen*) for Ginseng. If Ginseng is not available, one can use Radix Pseudostellariae (*Tai Zi Shen*) instead.

B. Bu Zhong Yi Qi Tang (Supplement the Center, Boost the Qi Decoction)

Composition:

Radix Astragali Membranacei (*Huang Qi*), 15g

Radix Glycyrrhizae (*Gan Cao*), 5g, mix-fried
Radix Panacis Ginseng (*Ren Shen*), 10g
Radix Angelicae Sinensis (*Dang Gui*), 10g
Pericarpium Citri Reticulatae (*Ju Pi*), 6g, remove the white
Rhizoma Cimicifugae (*Sheng Ma*), 3g
Radix Bupleuri (*Chai Hu*), 3g
Rhizoma Atractylodis Macrocephalae (*Bai Zhu*), 10g

Functions: Supplements the center and boosts the qi, upbears yang and lifts the fallen

Indications: 1) Spleen/stomach qi vacuity, 2) qi vacuity downward falling. Debility after prolonged disease, common cold in a person with bodily vacuity, chronic bronchitis, prolapsed uterus, prolapsed rectum, chronic hemorrhoids, gastroptosis, hernia, chronic gonorrhea, diarrhea, persistent malaria, habitual miscarriage, functional uterine bleeding and other hemorrhagic disorders, abnormal vaginal discharge, various postpartum problems, such as urinary incontinence, lochioschesis, and agalactia, chronic hepatitis, peritonitis, tuberculosis, neurasthenia, impotence, corneal ulcers, cerebral arteriosclerosis, pernicious anemia, leukopenia, chronic nephritis, and myasthenia gravis

Main signs & symptoms: 1) Fever, spontaneous sweating, thirst with a desire for warm drinks, shortness of breath, disinclination to speak, dyspnea on minor movement, bodily fatigue and chilled extremities, an ashen white or faded yellow facial color, loose stools, a pale tongue with thin white coating, and a flooding, vacuous or large, vacuous pulse; 2) anal prolapse, first and second degree uterine prolapse, prolonged diarrhea, prolonged dysentery, prolonged malaria, and other such complaints due to downward falling of clear yang

Contraindications:

1. Do not use for fever due to yin vacuity.

2. Only use for prolapse due to central qi vacuity.

Formula explanation:

Within this formula, Astragalus, which boosts the qi, is the sovereign. Ginseng, Atractylodis, and mix-fried Licorice fortify the spleen and boost the qi. They are the ministers. Together, they are able to supplement the center and boost the qi. Orange Peel is added to rectify the qi. *Dang Gui* is added to supplement the blood. These two are the assistant medicinals. Bupleurum and Cimicifugae upbear and lift downfallen clear yang. Thus they are the messengers within this qi-supplementing formula.

Additions & subtractions:

If blood vacuity is prominent, increase the dosage of *Dang Gui*.

For prolapse, increase the dosage of Astragalus and add Fructus Immaturus Citri Seu Ponciri (*Zhi Shi*).

For uterine prolapse, add Fructus Alpiniae Oxyphyllae (*Yi Zhi Ren*), Folium Artemisiae Argyii (*Ai Ye*), and Fructus Schizandrae Chinensis (*Wu Wei Zi*).

For abdominal pain, increase the dosage of mix-fried Licorice and add Radix Albus Paeoniae Lactiflorae (*Bai Shao*).

For more serious aversion to cold, add Cortex Cinnamomi (*Rou Gui*).

For headache with vertigo and dizziness, add Rhizoma Ligustici Wallichii (*Chuan Xiong*) and Rhizoma Pinelliae Ternatae (*Ban Xia*).

For pronounced headache, add Fructus Viticis (*Man Jing Zi*). If it becomes even more severe, add Rhizoma Ligustici Wallichii (*Chuan Xiong*).

For headache at the vertex or pain inside the head, add Radix Et Rhizoma Ligustici Chinensis (*Gao Ben*).

For severe headache, add Herba Cum Radice Asari (*Xi Xin*).

For vertigo and vomiting, add Radix Puerariae Lobatae (*Ge Gen*) and Rhizoma Alismatis (*Ze Xie*).

For bodily pain or a sensation of bodily heaviness, add *Wu Ling San* (Five *Ling* Powder) with Cinnamon subtracted.

For bodily heaviness, joint pain, irritability, loss of appetite, chest oppression, shortness of the breath, etc., replace Rhizoma Atractylodis Macrocephalae with Rhizoma Atractylodis (*Cang Zhu*), subtract *Dang Gui*, and add Radix Albus Paeoniae Lactiflorae (*Bai Shao*). This results in *Tiao Zhong Yi Qi Tang* (Regulate the Center, Boost the Qi Decoction).

For myasthenia gravis, increase the dosages of Astragalus and Cimicifuga.

For diarrhea due to excessive thinking and worry, add Radix Saussureae Seu Vladimiriae (*Mu Xiang*).

For diarrhea, subtract *Dang Gui* and add Sclerotium Poriae Cocos (*Fu Ling*), Rhizoma Atractylodis (*Cang Zhu*), and Fructus Alpiniae Oxyphyllae (*Yi Zhi Ren*).

Prolonged diarrhea with loss of securing and astringency, add Fructus Terminaliae Chebulae (*He Zi*), Semen Myristicae Fragrantis (*Rou Dou Kou*), Fructus Schizandrae Chinensis (*Wu Wei Zi*), and Fructus Pruni Mume (*Wu Mei*).

For dysentery with tenesmus, subtract *Dang Gui* and add Radix Saussureae Seu Vladimiriae (*Mu Xiang*).

For dysentery after the blood and pus have resolved but there is still foamy mucus, add blast-fried Rhizoma Zingiberis (*Pao Jiang*) and Hallyositum Rubrum (*Chi Shi Zhi*).

After dysentery when there is still tenesmus and mucus in the stools but constipation, add Radix Ledebouriellae Sesloidis (*Fang Feng*).

For cold stomach with qi stagnation, add Pericarpium Viridis Citri Reticulatae (*Qing Pi*), Fructus Amomi (*Sha Ren*), Radix Saussureae Seu Vladimiriae (*Mu Xiang*), and Fructus Alpiniae Oxyphyllae (*Yi Zhi Ren*).

For ringing in the ears or loss of hearing due to qi vacuity, add Fructus Corni Officinalis (*Shan Zhu Yu*) and Fructus Alpiniae Oxyphyllae (*Yi Zhi Ren*).

For diminished eyesight or blurred vision, add Fructus Lycii Chinensis (*Gou Qi Zi*) and Rhizoma Ligustici Wallichii (*Chuan Xiong*).

For habitual miscarriage, add Cortex Eucommiae Ulmoidis (*Du Zhong*) and Semen Cuscutae (*Tu Si Zi*).

For restless fetus and threatened abortion, add Gelatinum Corii Asini (*E Jiao*), and Folium Artemisiae Argyii (*Ai Ye*). This results in *Jia Jian Bu Zhong Yi Qi Tang* (Modified Supplement the Center, Boost the Qi Decoction). It can then be made even stronger by adding Radix Dipsaci (*Chuan Duan*) and Ramus Loranthi Seu Visci (*Sang Ji Sheng*).

For abnormal vaginal discharge, add *Er Miao San* (Two Wonders Powder), *i.e.*, Rhizoma Atractylodis (*Cang Zhu*) and Cortex Phello-dendri (*Huang Bai*).

For abdominal distention, add Fructus Immaturus Citri Seu Ponciri (*Zhi Shi*), Cortex Magnoliae Officinalis (*Hou Po*), Radix Saussureae Seu Vladimiriae (*Mu Xiang*), and Fructus Amomi (*Sha Ren*).

For *shan* or hernial disorders, add Semen Citri (*Ju He*), Fructus Foeniculi Vulgaris (*Xiao Hui Xiang*), and Semen Litchi Chinensis (*Li Zhi He*).

For constipation, add processed Radix Et Rhizoma Rhei (*Zhi Da Huang*).

For constipation due to spleen vacuity, add Honey (*Mi Tang*) and Sesame Oil (*Xiang You*).

For painful urinary strangury in the elderly due to fallen yang qi, add Rhizoma Alismatis (*Ze Xie*) and Caulis Akebiae Mutong (*Mu Tong*).

For taxation urinary strangury, add *Zhi Bai Di Huang Wan* (Anemarrhena & Phellodendron Rehmanniae Pills), *i.e.*, Rhizoma Anemarrhena (*Zhi Mu*), Cortex Phellodendri (*Huang Bai*), prepared Radix Rehmanniae (*Shu Di*), Radix Dioscoreae Oppositae (*Shan Yao*), Fructus Corni Officinalis (*Shan Zhu Yu*), Sclerotium Poriae Cocos (*Fu Ling*), Rhizoma Alismatis (*Ze Xie*), and Cortex Radicis Moutan (*Dan Pi*).

Also for taxation strangury, add *Liu Wei Di Huang Wan* (Six Flavors Rehmannia Pills), *i.e.* prepared Radix Rehmanniae (*Shu Di*), Radix Dioscoreae Oppositae (*Shan Yao*), Fructus Corni Officinalis (*Shan Zhu Yu*), Sclerotium Poriae Cocos (*Fu Ling*), Rhizoma Alismatis (*Ze Xie*), and Cortex Radicis Moutan (*Dan Pi*), plus Tuber Ophiopogonis Japonicae (*Mai Dong*) and Fructus Schizandrae Chinensis (*Wu Wei Zi*).

For frequent urination aggravated by exertion, add Radix Dioscoreae Oppositae (*Shan Yao*) and Fructus Schizandrae Chinensis (*Wu Wei Zi*).

103

For yellow urination after diarrhea, add Tuber Ophiopogonis Japonicae (*Mai Dong*) and Fructus Schizandrae Chinensis (*Wu Wei Zi*).

For premenstrual diarrhea, add blast-fried Rhizoma Zingiberis (*Pao Jiang*) and Rhizoma Coptidis Chinensis (*Huang Lian*).

For pediatric bed-wetting, add Ootheca Mantidis (*Sang Piao Xiao*) and Fructus Alpiniae Oxyphyllae (*Yi Zhi Ren*).

For chronic rhinitis, add Fructus Xanthii (*Cang Er Zi*) and Flos Magnoliae (*Xin Yi Hua*).

For corneal ulcers, add Scapus Eriocaulonis Buergeriani (*Gu Jing Cao*), Semen Cassiae Torae (*Jue Ming Zi*), and Radix Dioscoreae Oppositae (*Shan Yao*).

If there is concomitant yin vacuity, either subtract Bupleurum and Cimicifugae or reduce their dosages and add Rhizoma Anemarrhenae (*Zhi Mu*) and Cortex Phellodendri (*Huang Bai*).

Also for yin vacuity, subtract Cimicifuga and Bupleurum and add Fructus Corni Officinalis (*Shan Zhu Yu*), Radix Dioscoreae Oppositae (*Shan Yao*), and prepared Radix Rehmanniae (*Shu Di*).

For qi vacuity fever, add Rhizoma Anemarrhenae (*Zhi Mu*) and Cortex Radicis Lycii (*Di Gu Pi*).

Also for qi vacuity fever, increase the dosage of Bupleurum and add Radix Scutellariae Baicalensis (*Huang Qin*) and Radix Puerariae Lobatae (*Ge Gen*).

For coronary heart disease with exertional angina pectoris, add Radix Salviae Miltiorrhizae (*Dan Shen*), Rhizoma Ligustici Wallichii (*Chuan Xiong*), Radix Rubrus Paeoniae Lactiflorae (*Chi Shao*), Flos Carthami

Tinctorii (*Hong Hua*), and Lignum Dalbergiae Odoriferae (*Jiang Xiang*).

If there is lung heat, subtract Ginseng.

For sore throat, add Radix Platycodi Grandiflori (*Jie Geng*).

For excessive menstruation, add wine-fried Radix Albus Paeoniae Lactiflorae (*Jiu Chao Bai Shao*). If there is liver heat, add Radix Scutellariae Baicalensis (*Huang Qin*).

For functional uterine bleeding, *i.e.*, *beng lou*, add Radix Sanguisorbae (*Di Yu*) for damp or replete heat, Folium Artemisiae Argyii (*Ai Ye*) and Gelatinum Corii Asini (*E Jiao*) for qi vacuity, raw Radix Rehmanniae (*Sheng Di*) for vacuity heat, and Os Sepiae Seu Sepiellae (*Hai Piao Xiao*) for loss of securing and astringing.

For excessive menstruation or uterine bleeding with pale, watery blood and accompanied by palpitations, shortness of breath, slow speech, fatigue, and a dragging feeling in the lower abdomen, subtract *Dang Gui*, Bupleurum, and Orange Peel. This results in *Ju Yuan Jian* (Lift the Source Decoction). This formula can then be augmented by adding Os Sepiae Seu Sepiellae (*Hai Piao Xiao*), Radix Rubiae Cordifoliae (*Qian Cao*), and Fructus Pruni Mume (*Wu Mei*). If there is liver heat, add Radix Scutellariae Baicalensis (*Huang Qin*).

For numbness of the fingers and face due to qi vacuity with exuberant wind, subtract *Dang Gui*, Atractylodis, and Orange Peel, and add Radix Albus Paeoniae Lactiflorae (*Bai Shao*) and Fructus Schizandrae Chinensis (*Wu Wei Zi*).

For numbness accompanying bodily weakness, dry, flaky skin, and itching, add prepared Radix Rehmanniae (*Shu Di*) and Radix Albus Paeoniae Lactiflorae (*Bai Shao*).

For neurasthenia, add Os Draconis (*Long Gu*), Concha Ostreae (*Mu Li*), and Caulis Polygoni Multiflori (*Ye Jiao Teng*).

6.2 *Bu Xue Ji* (Blood-supplementing formulas)

Representative formulas:

A. *Si Wu Tang* (Four Materials Decoction)

Composition:

Radix Angelicae Sinensis (*Dang Gui*), 10g, stir-fried in wine
Rhizoma Ligustici Wallichii (*Chuan Xiong*), 8g
Radix Albus Paeoniae Lactiflorae (*Bai Shao*), 12g
prepared dry Radix Rehmanniae (*Shu Gan Di Huang*), 12g

Functions: Supplements the blood and regulates the blood

Indications: *Chong* and *ren* vacuity detriment, menstruation not regulated, lower abdominal pain, flooding and leaking. Dysmenorrhea, irregular menstruation, uterine bleeding, anemia due to various causes, threatened miscarriage, abdominal pain during pregnancy, postpartum weakness, scanty lactation, hemafecia, dry skin, constipation, and neurogenic headache

Main signs & symptoms: Dizziness, tinnitus, palpitations, loss of sleep, blurred vision, lusterless facial complexion and nails, generalized muscular tension, irregular menstruation with scant flow or blood lumps and clots, possible amenorrhea, occasional aching and pain, restless fetus during pregnancy, downward precipitation of blood which will not stop, postpartum lochia which will not stop, abdominal masses, lower abdominal dragging pain, occasional fever and chills, a pale tongue, and a wiry, fine or fine, choppy pulse

Contraindications:

1. Do not use for severe anemia or blood loss. In that case, boost the qi in order to supplement the blood.
2. Do not use if there is spleen and stomach vacuity and dampness with poor appetite and loose stools.

Formula explanation:

In this formula, *Dang Gui* supplements the blood and quickens the blood. Prepared Rehmannia supplements the blood. These two are the rulers. Ligusticum enters the blood division where it rectifies the qi within the blood. Peony restrains yin and nourishes the blood. Thus all the ingredients in this formula are categorized as blood division medicinals.

Additions & subtractions:

To quicken the blood and transform stasis, replace prepared Rehmannia with raw Radix Rehmanniae (*Sheng Di*) and White Peony with Radix Rubrus Paeoniae Lactiflorae (*Chi Shao*).

Or for blood heat, replace White Peony with Red Peony and for stasis, replace prepared Rehmannia with raw Rehmannia.

For severe blood stasis with abdominal pain, add Semen Pruni Persicae (*Tao Ren*) and Flos Carthami Tinctorii (*Hong Hua*). This results in *Tao Hong Si Wu Tang* (Persica & Carthamus Four Materials Decoction).

Also for blood stasis, add *Gui Zhi Fu Ling Wan* (Cinnamon & Poria Pills), *i.e.*, Ramulus Cinnamomi (*Gui Zhi*), Radix Rubrus Paeoniae Lactiflorae (*Chi Shao*), Cortex Radicis Moutan (*Dan Pi*), and Sclerotium Poriae Cocos (*Fu Ling*).

For qi stagnation with abdominal distention, add Radix Linderae Strychnifoliae (*Wu Yao*) and Rhizoma Cyperi Rotundi (*Xiang Fu*).

For postpartum uterine bleeding or fetal leakage, *i.e.*, threatened abortion, add Folium Artemisiae Argyii (*Ai Ye*) and Gelatinum Corii Asini (*E Jiao*). This results in *Jiao Ai Tang* (Donkey Skin Glue & Artemisia Argyium Decoction).

For dysmenorrhea due to both blood stasis and vacuity, add Herba Leonuri Heterophylli (*Yi Mu Cao*), Rhizoma Cyperi Rotundi (*Xiang Fu*), and Rhizoma Corydalis Yanhusuo (*Yan Hu*).

For qi vacuity with shortness of breath and irregular menstruation with excessive blood, add Radix Panacis Ginseng (*Ren Shen*) and Radix Astragali Membranacei (*Huang Qi*). This results in *Sheng Yu Tang* (Sage-like Healing Decoction).

With accompanying cold signs and symptoms, add Cortex Cinnamomi (*Rou Gui*) and blast-fried Rhizoma Zingiberis (*Pao Jiang*). This results in *Jiang Gui Si Wu Tang* (Ginger & Cinnamon Four Materials Decoction).

With accompanying heat signs and symptoms, add Radix Scutellariae Baicalensis (*Huang Qin*) and Fructus Gardeniae Jasminoidis (*Zhi Zi*).

For even more severe heat, add Scutellaria plus Rhizoma Coptidis Chinensis (*Huang Lian*) and Cortex Phellodendri (*Huang Bai*). This results in *San Huang Si Wu Tang* (Three Yellow Four Materials Decoction).

For yet more heat, add Scutellaria, Coptis, Phellodendron, and Gardenia. This results in *Wen Qing Yin* (Warming & Clearing Decoction). This formula is used to treat both excessive uterine bleeding and also recalcitrant skin diseases.

Again for blood vacuity complicated by heat, add Radix Scutellariae Baicalensis (*Huang Qin*), Rhizoma Coptidis Chinensis (*Huang Lian*), and Tuber Ophiopogonis Japonicae (*Mai Dong*). This results in *Qin Lian Si Wu Tang* (Scutellaria & Coptis Four Materials Decoction).

For yin vacuity night sweats, add Radix Astragali Membranacei (*Huang Qi*), Rhizoma Coptidis Chinensis (*Huang Lian*), Radix Scutellariae Baicalensis (*Huang Qin*), and Cortex Phellodendri (*Huang Bai*). This results in *Dang Gui Liu Huang Tang* (*Dang Gui* Six Yellows Decoction).

For liver blood and yin vacuity with blurred vision, headache, dizziness, dry eyes, photophobia, easy anger, numbness, muscle twitching, malar flushing, a dry, red tongue, and a wiry, fine, rapid pulse, add Semen Zizyphi Spinosae (*Suan Zao Ren*), Fructus Chaenomelis Lagenariae (*Mu Gua*), and mix-fried Radix Glycyrrhizae (*Zhi Gan Cao*). This results in *Bu Gan Tang* (Supplement the Liver Decoction).

For amenorrhea due to blood stasis and replete heat in the interior with dry, hard stools and constipation, add Radix Et Rhizoma Rhei (*Da Huang*), Mirabilitum (*Mang Xiao*), and Radix Glycyrrhizae (*Gan Cao*). This results in *Yu Zhu San* (Jade Candle Powder).

For threatened abortion, add Radix Scutellariae Baicalensis (*Huang Qin*) and Rhizoma Atractylodis Macrocephalae (*Bai Zhu*).

For infertility, habitual miscarriage, and other disorders of pregnancy, subtract prepared Rehmannia and add Rhizoma Atractylodis Macrocephalae (*Bai Zhu*), Sclerotium Poriae Cocos (*Fu Ling*), and Rhizoma Alismatis (*Ze Xie*). This results in *Dang Gui Shao Yao San* (*Dang Gui* & Peony Powder).

For cold pain and distention in the lower abdomen with a pale tongue and white coating during the second and third trimesters of pregnancy, add Rhizoma Cyperi Rotundi (*Xiang Fu*), Folium Artemisiae Argyii (*Ai Ye*), Radix Astragali Membranacei (*Huang Qi*), Fructus Evodiae

Rutecarpae (*Wu Zhu Yu*), Cortex Cinnamomi (*Rou Gui*), and Radix Dipsaci (*Xu Duan*). This results in *Ai Fu Nuan Gong Wan* (Artemisia Argyium & Cyperus Warm the Palace [*i.e.,* Uterus] Decoction).

For atony with weakness of the limbs and difficulty moving due to a combination of damp heat, spleen vacuity, and liver and kidney vacuity, add Tuber Ophiopogonis Japonicae (*Mai Dong*), Cortex Phellodendri (*Huang Bai*), Rhizoma Atractylodis (*Cang Zhu*), Cortex Eucommiae Ulmoidis (*Du Zhong*), Fructus Schizandrae Chinensis (*Wu Wei Zi*), Radix Panacis Ginseng (*Ren Shen*), Rhizoma Coptidis Chinensis (*Huang Lian*), Rhizoma Anemarrhenae (*Zhi Mu*), and Radix Achyranthis Bidentatae (*Niu Xi*). This results in *Jia Wei Si Wu Tang* (Added Flavors Four Materials Decoction).

For leukopenia and thrombocytopenia due to radiation or chemotherapy, subtract Ligusticum and add Arillus Euphoriae Longanae (*Long Yan Rou*), Radix Salviae Miltiorrhizae (*Dan Shen*), and Caulis Millettiae Seu Spatholobi (*Ji Xue Teng*). This results in *Dang Gui Ji Xue Teng Tang* (*Dang Gui* & Millettia Decoction).

For anemia and heart palpitations, add Cortex Cinnamomi (*Rou Gui*), Sclerotium Poriae Cocos (*Fu Ling*), Rhizoma Atractylodis Macrocephalae (*Bai Zhu*), and Radix Glycyrrhizae (*Gan Cao*). This results in *Lian Zhu Yin* (Lotus & Pearl Drink).

For over 100 more modifications of *Si Wu Tang*, see my *How to Write a TCM Herbal Formula*, Blue Poppy Press, Boulder, CO, 1993.

B. *Gui Pi Tang* (Restore the Spleen Decoction)

Composition:

Radix Panacis Ginseng (*Ren Shen*), 6g
Radix Astragali Membranacei (*Huang Qi*), 12g

Rhizoma Atractylodis Macrocephalae (*Bai Zhu*), 9g
Sclerotium Pararadicis Poriae Cocos (*Fu Shen*), 9g
Arillus Euphoriae Longanae (*Long Yan Rou*), 12g
Semen Zizyphi Spinosae (*Suan Zao Ren*), 12g
Radix Saussureae Seu Vladimiriae (*Mu Xiang*), 6g
Radix Glycyrrhizae (*Gan Cao*), 6g, mix-fried
Radix Angelicae Sinensis (*Dang Gui*), 9g
Radix Polygalae Tenuifoliae (*Yuan Zhi*), 9g
raw Rhizoma Zingiberis (*Sheng Jiang*), 3g
Fructus Zizyphi Jujubae (*Da Zao*), 5 pieces

Functions: Boosts the qi and supplements the blood, fortifies the spleen and nourishes the heart

Indications: 1) Heart/spleen dual vacuity, taxation damage of the heart and spleen, qi and blood insufficiency, 2) spleen not gathering the blood. Neurasthenia, gastric and duodenal ulcers, functional uterine bleeding, thrombocytopenic purpura, aplastic anemia, common anemia, chronic hemorrhagic disorders, menorrhagia, post-concussion syndrome, myasthenia gravis, congestive heart disease, supraventricular tachycardia, palpitations, cervicitis, uterine cancer, leukemia, insomnia, poor memory, genital itching, nocturnal emission, impotence, and chronic gonorrhea

Main signs & symptoms: 1) Heart palpitations, poor memory, insomnia, night sweats, vacuity heat (*i.e.*, feverishness), diminished appetite, bodily fatigue, a faded yellow facial color, a pale, fat tongue with thin, white coating, and a fine, relaxed/retarded or fine, weak pulse; 2) hemafecia, uterine bleeding, early periods, excessive menstruation but pale colored blood or dribbling and dripping which will not stop, or abnormal vaginal discharge

Formula explanation:

In this formula, Ginseng, Astragalus, Licorice, Ginger, and Red Dates are all sweet and warm and supplement the spleen and boost the qi. *Dang Gui* is sweet and acrid. It warms and nourishes the liver and generates heart blood. Spirit of Poria, Zizyphus Spinosa, and Longans are sweet and neutral. They nourish the heart and quiet the spirit. Polygala joins and frees the flow between the heart and kidneys. It also stabilizes the will (or orientations, *i.e.*, emotions) and tranquilizes the heart. Saussurea rectifies the qi and arouses the spleen. This ingredient is added because qi-boosting, blood-supplementing formulas use enriching, greasy ingredients which may stagnate the qi and hinder the spleen and stomach's function of transportation and transformation.

Additions & subtractions:

For vacuous patients who cannot take large supplementing decoctions without experiencing abdominal distention and fullness, add Pericarpium Citri Reticulatae (*Chen Pi*) and Fructus Amomi (*Sha Ren*).

For more severe fatigue and spontaneous sweating, increase the dosage of Astragalus.

To augment this formula's ability to nourish the blood, add prepared Radix Rehmanniae (*Shu Di*).

For anemia, add Rhizoma Ligustici Wallichii (*Chuan Xiong*) and Radix Albus Paeoniae Lactiflorae (*Bai Shao*).

For painful menstruation containing clots, add Tuber Curcumae (*Yu Jin*) and Rhizoma Cyperi Rotundi (*Xiang Fu*).

For blackish menstrual blood, add Flos Carthami Tinctorii (*Hong Hua*), Cortex Radicis Moutan (*Dan Pi*), and Fructus Gardeniae Jasminoidis (*Shan Zhi Zi*).

For uterine bleeding which is excessive in amount but pale in color and thin in consistency, add Gelatinum Corii Asini (*E Jiao*), Ramus Loranthi Seu Visci (*Sang Ji Sheng*), and Radix Polygoni Multiflori (*He Shou Wu*).

For prolonged bleeding, add Gelatinum Corii Asini (*E Jiao*), Folium Artemisiae Argyii (*Ai Ye*), and Gelatinum Cornu Cervi (*Lu Jiao Jiao*).

For profuse uterine bleeding which is cold in nature, add Folium Artemisiae Argyii (*Ai Ye*), blast-fried Rhizoma Zingiberis (*Pao Jiang*), Crinis Carbonisatus (*Xue Yu Tan*), and Fructus Schizandrae Chinensis (*Wu Wei Zi*).

For metrorrhagia due to the spleen failing to control the blood, subtract Saussurea and Polygala and add Fructus Corni Officinalis (*Shan Zhu Yu*).

For flooding (*beng*) which suddenly changes to leaking (*lou*), add Fructus Corni Officinalis (*Shan Zhu Yu*) and Fructus Schizandrae Chinensis (*Wu Wei Zi*).

For numbness in the upper extremities, add Radix Et Rhizoma Notopterygii (*Qiang Huo*) and Rhizoma Ligustici Wallichii (*Chuan Xiong*).

For numbness in the lower back and lower extremities, add Radix Clematidis (*Wei Ling Xian*), Radix Angelicae Pubescentis (*Du Huo*), and Radix Achyranthis Bidentatae (*Niu Xi*).

For low back aching and weakness, add Ramus Loranthi Seu Visci (*Sang Ji Sheng*), Fructus Lycii Chinensis (*Gou Qi Zi*), and Radix Polygoni Multiflori (*He Shou Wu*) or Radix Achyranthis Bidentatae (*Niu Xi*) and Polygonum Multiflorum.

For indigestion with abdominal distention and fullness, add Massa Medica Fermentata (*Shen Qu*), Fructus Germinatus Hordei Vulgaris (*Mai Ya*), and Fructus Crataegi (*Shan Zha*).

For edema, add Semen Coicis Lachryma-jobi (*Yi Ren*) and Rhizoma Alismatis (*Ze Xie*).

For insomnia and neurosis, add Semen Biotae Orientalis (*Bai Zi Ren*).

For concomitant liver depression and constipation, add Radix Bupleuri (*Chai Hu*) and Fructus Gardeniae Jasminoidis (*Zhi Zi*).

If there is simultaneous blood stasis in the lower abdomen, add Rhizoma Ligustici Wallichii (*Chuan Xiong*), Radix Achyranthis Bidentatae (*Niu Xi*), and Cortex Radicis Moutan (*Dan Pi*).

For fallen qi, add Radix Bupleuri (*Chai Hu*) and Rhizoma Cimicifugae (*Sheng Ma*).

For chronic cough, add Fructus Schizandrae Chinensis (*Wu Wei Zi*) and Rhizoma Pinelliae Ternatae (*Ban Xia*).

For bloody stools due to spleen vacuity, subtract Polygala and add blast-fried Rhizoma Zingiberis (*Pao Jiang*).

For premenstrual headache complicated by liver qi, add Rhizoma Cyperi Rotundi (*Xiang Fu*), Radix Albus Paeoniae Lactiflorae (*Bai Shao*), Fructus Tribuli Terrestris (*Bai Ji Li*), and Radix Bupleuri (*Chai Hu*).

Comment: For the treatment of aplastic anemia, this formula may be used with Western medicinals and blood transfusions.

6.3 *Bu Yin Ji* (Yin-supplementing formulas)

Representative formula: *Liu Wei Di Huang Wan* (Six Flavors Rehmannia Pills)

Composition:

prepared Radix Rehmanniae (*Shu Di Huang*), 24g
Fructus Corni Officinalis (*Shan Zhu Yu*), 12g
dry Radix Dioscoreae Oppositae (*Gan Shan Yao*), 12g
Rhizoma Alismatis (*Ze Xie*), 9g
Sclerotium Poriae Cocos (*Fu Ling*), 9g
Cortex Radicis Moutan (*Dan Pi*), 9g

Functions: Enriches and supplements the liver and kidneys

Indications: Liver/kidney yin vacuity. Retarded growth of children, lumbago, optic neuritis, central retinitis, optic nerve atrophy, pulmonary tuberculosis, diabetes, hyperthyroidism, Addison's disease, hypertension, neurasthenia, functional uterine bleeding, chronic urinary tract infection, chronic nephritis, chronic glomerulonephritis, nephroatrophy, deafness, impotence, nocturnal emission, nocturia, menopause, senility

Main signs & symptoms: Low back and knee soreness and weakness, dizziness and vertigo, tinnitus and deafness, night sweats and spermatorrhea, bone-steaming and tidal fevers, heat in the hands, feet, and heart (or heat in the centers of the hands and feet), wasting thirst, possible vacuity fire toothache, dry mouth and throat, a red tongue with scant coating, and a thready, rapid pulse

Contraindications:

1. Use with care in patients with a white, slimy tongue coating and indigestion indicating spleen vacuity and dampness or food stagnation.
2. Do not use in patients with diarrhea.

Formula explanation:

Within this formula, prepared Rehmannia is the sovereign ingredient. It enriches kidney yin and boosts the essence and marrow. Cornus assists in warming and enriching the kidneys and boosting the liver. Dioscorea enriches the kidneys and supplements the spleen. These are the three yin-supplementing medicinals in this formula. They are called the *san bu* or three supplementers. These are then combined with three draining or opening ingredients called the *san xie*, the three drainers. Alisma aids Rehmannia by draining any exuberance of kidney fire and downbears turbidity. Moutan aids Cornus by draining liver fire. In addition, it quickens the blood and transforms stasis. Since this formula is so often used in the elderly and the chronically ill, an element of blood stasis is often found in cases for whom this formula is appropriate. Poria assists Dioscorea by percolating spleen dampness. Further, Poria and Alisma work together to eliminate dampness and disinhibit water.

Additions & subtractions:

For dry, red eyes or blurred vision, add Flos Chrysanthemi Morifolii (*Ju Hua*) and Fructus Lycii Chinensis (*Gou Qi Zi*). This results in *Qi Ju Di Huang Wan* (Lycium & Chrysanthemum Rehmannia Pills).

For wheezing and shortness of breath on slight movement, add Fructus Schizandrae Chinensis (*Wu Wei Zi*). This results in *Du Qi Wan* (Capital Qi Pills).

Also for wheezing and chronic cough due to lung/kidney yin vacuity, add Schizandra and Tuber Ophiopogonis Japonicae (*Mai Dong*). This results in *Mai Wei Di Huang Wan* (Ophiopogon & Schizandra Rehmannia Pills). This is also called *Ba Xian Chang Shou Wan* (Eight Immortals Long Life Pills).

For extreme yin vacuity, add Tuber Ophiopogonis Japonicae (*Mai Men Dong*), Tuber Asparagi Cochinensis (*Tian Men Dong*), and Radix Scrophulariae Ningpoensis (*Xuan Shen*).

For yin vacuity with exuberant fire, add Rhizoma Anemarrhenae (*Zhi Mu*) and Cortex Phellodendri (*Huang Bai*). This results in *Zhi Bai Di Huang Wan* (Anemarrhena & Phellodendron Rehmannia Pills).

For severe night sweats, add Semen Cuscutae (*Tu Si Zi*) and Stamen Nelumbinis Nuciferae (*Lian Xu*).

For slow physical and mental development, add Cornu Cervi Parvum (*Lu Rong*), Cortex Radicis Acanthopanacis (*Wu Jia Pi*), Secretio Moschi Moschiferi (*She Xiang*). This results in *Jia Wei Liu Wei Di Huang Wan* (Added Flavors Rehmannia Pills).

For tinnitus, deafness, dizziness and vertigo, and blurred vision, add Magnetitum (*Ci Shi*), Rhizoma Acori Graminei (*Shi Chang Pu*), and Fructus Schizandrae Chinensis (*Wu Wei Zi*). This results in *Er Long Zuo Ci Wan* (Pill for Deafness that is Kind to the Left [Kidney]).

For scanty menstruation and/or chronic dry eczema, add Radix Angelicae Sinensis (*Dang Gui*). This results in *Dang Gui Di Huang Yin* (*Dang Gui* & Rehmannia Drink).

Also for scanty menstruation, add *Dang Gui* and Radix Albus Paeoniae Lactiflorae (*Bai Shao*). This results in *Gui Shao Di Huang Wan* (*Dang Gui* & Peony Rehmannia Pills).

117

For postpartum continuous sweating, add Fructus Schizandrae Chinensis (*Wu Wei Zi*) and mix-fried Radix Astragali Membranacei (*Zhi Huang Qi*). This results in *Ba Wei Di Huang Wan* (Eight Flavors Rehmannia Pills).

For blurred vision due to liver/kidney vacuity, add raw Radix Rehmanniae (*Sheng Di*), Radix Bupleuri (*Chai Hu*), Radix Angelicae Sinensis (*Dang Gui*), and Fructus Schizandrae Chinensis (*Wu Wei Zi*). This results in *Ming Mu Di Huang Wan* (Eye-brightening Rehmannia Pills).

For diabetes mellitus, add Radix Trichosanthis Kirlowii (*Tian Hua Fen*).

If there is liver/kidney dual vacuity with concomitant liver depression, add *Xiao Yao San* (Rambling Powder), *i.e.*, Radix Bupleuri (*Chai Hu*), Rhizoma Atractylodis Macrocephalae (*Bai Zhu*), Sclerotium Poriae Cocos (*Fu Ling*), Radix Angelicae Sinensis (*Dang Gui*), Radix Albus Paeoniae Lactiflorae (*Bai Shao*), and mix-fried Radix Glycyrrhizae (*Zhi Gan Cao*).

If there is depressive heat, add *Dan Zhi Xiao Yao San, i.e., Xiao Yao San* as above plus Cortex Radicis Moutan (*Dan Pi*) and Fructus Gardeniae Jasminoidis (*Shan Zhi Yi*).

For extreme thirst due to stomach heat, add Gypsum (*Shi Gao*) and Herba Dendrobii (*Shi Hu*).

For liver/gallbladder heat with a bitter taste in the mouth, fever and chills, low fever, possible hepatitis, and burning urination, add Radix Bupleuri (*Chai Hu*), Radix Scutellariae Baicalensis (*Huang Qin*), and Fructus Gardeniae Jasminoidis (*Zhi Zi*).

6.4 *Bu Yang Ji* (Yang-supplementing formulas)

Representative formulas:

A. *Jin Gui Shen Qi Wan* (Golden Cabinet Kidney Qi Pills)

Composition:

prepared Radix Rehmanniae (*Shu Di*), 25g
Fructus Corni Officinalis (*Shan Zhu Yu*), 12g
Radix Dioscoreae Oppositae (*Shan Yao*), 15g
Rhizoma Alismatis (*Ze Xie*), 9g
Sclerotium Poriae Cocos (*Fu Ling*), 12g
Cortex Radicis Moutan (*Dan Pi*), 9g
Ramulus Cinnamomi (*Gui Zi*), 6g
Radix Praeparatus Aconiti Carmichaeli (*Fu Zi*), 9g

Functions: Warms and supplements kidney yang

Indications: Kidney yang insufficiency. Nephritis, nephrosclerosis, kidney stones, kidney tuberculosis, pyelitis, albuminuria, edema, cystitis, chronic urethritis, prostatic hypertrophy, urinary incontinence, diabetes, cerebral hemorrhage, arteriosclerosis, hypertension, hypotension, neurasthenia, spermatorrhea, impotence, lumbago, sciatica, beriberi, cataracts, glaucoma, decrease in eyesight, keratitis, eczema, senile pruritus, vaginal itching, urticaria, chronic gonorrhea, rectal prolapse, menopausal complaints, primary hyperaldosteronism, Addison's disease, hypothyroidism, postpartum urinary retention, arthritis, and chronic bronchial asthma

Main signs & symptoms: Low back pain, weak knees, a cold feeling in the lower half of the body, lower abdominal tension, inhibited urination or excessive urination, nocturia, cockcrow diarrhea, a pale, fat tongue with a thin, white, not dry coating, and a deep, fine pulse in the foot position

Contraindications:

1. Do not use in yin vacuity with a dry mouth and throat and a red tongue with scant coating unless there are cold feet below signifying concomitant yang vacuity.
2. Do not use in patients with chronic gastrointestinal weakness and diarrhea.

Formula explanation:

This formula uses prepared Rehmannia to enrich and supplement kidney yin. Cornus and Dioscorea enrich and supplement the liver and spleen, thus assisting the enrichment and supplementation of yin within the kidneys. A small amount of Cinnamon and Aconite are added to warm and supplement yang within the kidneys. Alisma and Poria disinhibit water and percolate dampness, while Moutan clears and drains liver fire. Thus this combination of medicinals warms and supplements kidney yang, supplements at the same time as it drains, and supplements without being greasy. It is also based on the notion of seeking yang within yin.

Additions & subtractions:

For cold feet, edema, tinnitus, deafness, dysuria, and low back pain, add Cornu Cervi Parvum (*Lu Rong*) and Fructus Schizandrae Chinensis (*Wu Wei Zi*). This results in *Shi Bu Wan* (Ten Supplements Pills).

If cold is more severe, replace Ramulus Cinnamomi with Cortex Cinnamomi (*Rou Gui*).

For nocturia, add Fructus Schizandrae Chinensis (*Wu Wei Zi*).

For frequent, long, clear urination and emaciation, add Fructus Psoraleae Corylifoliae (*Bu Gu Zhi*) and Cornu Cervi Parvum (*Lu Rong*).

For impotence, add Radix Morindae (*Ba Ji Rou*), Herba Cistanchis (*Rou Cong Rong*), Herba Cynomorii Songarici (*Suo Yang*), and Fructus Lycii Chinensis (*Gou Qi Zi*).

Also for impotence and premature ejaculation, add Herba Allii Fistulosi (*Cong Bai*), Semen Allii Tuberosi (*Jiu Zi*), Actinolitum (*Yang Qi Shi*), Herba Epimedii (*Yin Yang Huo*), and Rhizoma Curculiginis Orchoidis (*Xian Mao*).

For nocturnal emission and spermatorrhea, add Fructus Rosae Laevigatae (*Jin Ying Zi*), Stamen Nelumbinis Nuciferae (*Lian Xu*), Radix Polygalae Tenuifoliae (*Yuan Zhi*), Cortex Phellodendri (*Huang Bai*), Fructus Amomi (*Sha Ren*), and Radix Glycyrrhizae (*Gan Cao*).

For both male and female infertility, add Semen Cuscutae (*Tu Si Zi*), Radix Polygalae Tenuifoliae (*Yuan Zhi*), Fructus Lycii Chinensis (*Gou Qi Zi*), Fructus Psoraleae Corylifoliae (*Bu Gu Zhi*), Fructus Rubi (*Fu Pen Zi*), Herba Cistanchis (*Rou Cong Rong*), and Fructus Schizandrae Chinensis (*Wu Wei Zi*).

For painful urination due to cold in the lower burner with frequent, scanty urination, and terminal dribbling, add Cornu Cervi Parvum (*Lu Rong*) and Lignum Aquilariae Agallochae (*Chen Xiang*).

For incontinence or turbid urine after overusing bitter, cold medicinals, subtract Alisma and add Fructus Schizandrae Chinensis (*Wu Wei Zi*).

For edema in the lower extremities, add *Wu Pi Yin* (Five Peels Drink), *i.e.*, Cortex Sclerotii Poriae Cocos (*Fu Ling Pi*), Cortex Radicis Mori (*Sang Bai Pi*), Cortex Rhizomatis Zingiberis (*Sheng Jiang Pi*),

121

Pericarpium Arecae Catechu (*Da Fu Pi*), and Pericarpium Citri Reticulatae (*Chen Pi*).

For edema with abdominal bloating, extremely scant urination, and severe proteinuria, add or alternate with *Li Zhong Tang*, *i.e.*, Radix Panacis Ginseng (*Ren Shen*), Rhizoma Atractylodis Macrocephalae (*Bai Zhu*), dry Rhizoma Zingiberis (*Gan Jiang*), and mix-fried Radix Glycyrrhizae (*Zhi Gan Cao*).

For low back and knee soreness and weakness, add Radix Dipsaci (*Xu Duan*) and Cortex Eucommiae Ulmoidis (*Du Zhong*).

For nephritis with concomitant qi vacuity, add Radix Codonopsis Pilosulae (*Dang Shen*) and Radix Astragali Membranacei (*Huang Qi*).

For prostatitis with scanty urine in older men, replace Ramulus Cinnamomi with Cortex Cinnamomi (*Rou Gui*) and add Rhizoma Anemarrhenae (*Zhi Mu*) and Cortex Phellodendri (*Huang Bai*).

For edema and painful urination including prostatitis, add Radix Cyathulae (*Chuan Niu Xi*) and Semen Plantaginis (*Che Qian Zi*). This results in *Ji Sheng Shen Qi Wan* (Formulas for the Living Kidney Qi Pills).

For frequent urination which is not inhibited, subtract Alisma and Poria and add Radix Linderae Strychnifoliae (*Wu Yao*), Fructus Alpiniae Oxyphyllae (*Yi Zhi Ren*), Fructus Rubi (*Fu Pen Zi*), Os Draconis (*Long Gu*), and Concha Ostreae (*Mu Li*).

If there is cough with phlegm and severe asthma, add Hallyositum Rubrum (*Chi Shi*), Radix Panacis Ginseng (*Ren Shen*), and Fructus Schizandrae Chinensis (*Wu Wei Zi*).

For asthma with palpitations and dizziness, add Hallyositum Rubrum and Schizandra and increase the dosage of Poria.

For pain in the foot, sole, or heel, add Radix Achyranthis Bidentatae (*Niu Xi*) and Cornu Cervi Parvum (*Lu Rong*).

For upper back and spinal pain, add Rhizoma Cibotii Barometsis (*Gou Ji*) and Cornu Cervi Parvum (*Lu Rong*).

For hypertension, add Os Draconis (*Long Gu*) and Concha Ostreae (*Mu Li*).

For tinnitus, deafness, a pressure in the ears, add Spica Prunellae Vulgaris (*Xia Gu Cao*), Hallyositum Rubrum (*Chi Shi*), Radix Bupleuri (*Chai Hu*), Rhizoma Acori Graminei (*Shi Chang Pu*), and Radix Polygalae Tenuifoliae (*Yuan Zhi*).

For early stage cataracts with blurred vision, add Radix Et Rhizoma Notopterygii (*Qiang Huo*), Rhizoma Ligustici Wallichii (*Chuan Xiong*), Radix Bupleuri (*Chai Hu*), Radix Rubrus Paeoniae Lactiflorae (*Chi Shao*), and Concha Haliotidis (*Shi Jue Ming*).

For retinitis, add Scapus Eriocaulonis Buergeriani (*Gu Jing Cao*), Herba Equiseti Hiemalis (*Mu Zei Cao*), Semen Cassiae Torae (*Jue Ming Cao*), and Semen Celosiae Argenteae (*Qing Xiang Zi*).

For toothache, oral ulcers, and gingivitis, replace Ramulus Cinnamomi with Cortex Cinnamomi (*Rou Gui*) and add Rhizoma Coptidis Chinensis (*Huang Lian*).

For poor memory and hair loss, add Radix Polygoni Multiflori (*He Shou Wu*).

For prolapsed kidney or bladder, add or alternate with *Bu Zhong Yi Qi Tang*.

Comment: Although modern TCM texts say this formula is contraindicated for vacuity heat with sore throat, heat in the five hearts, etc., originally it was intended to treat the combination of vacuity heat in the upper burner with vacuity cold in the lower burner. If there are cold feet, this formula may be used with appropriate modifications even if there are signs of vacuity heat above.

B. *Er Xian Tang* (Two Immortals Decoction)

Composition:

Rhizoma Curculiginis Orchoidis (*Xian Mao*), 12g
Herba Epimedii (*Xian Ling Pi*), 12g
Radix Morindae (*Ba Ji Tian*), 9g
Radix Angelicae Sinensis (*Dang Gui*), 9g
Cortex Phellodendri (*Huang Bai*), 9g
Rhizoma Anemarrhenae (*Zhi Mu*), 9g

Functions: Enriches and supplements the liver and kidneys, warms yang but drains fire, regulates and harmonizes the *chong* and *ren*

Indications: Liver blood and kidney yin and yang vacuity, loss of harmony of the *chong* and *ren*. Menopausal complaints, amenorrhea, hypertension, nephritis, chronic pyelonephritis, chronic glomerulonephritis, polycystic kidneys, renal vascular disease, urinary tract infection, and hypofunction of the anterior pituitary

Main signs & symptoms: Irregular menstruation, dizziness, tinnitus, headache, soreness and weakness of the low back and knees, cold lower extremities, hot flashes, night sweats, irritability, insomnia, nocturia, frequent urination, a pale tongue with scant coating, and a fine, wiry, rapid, possibly floating pulse

Formula explanation:

Curculigo and Epimedium are the sovereign medicinals in this formula. Together with their minister, Morinda, they warm and supplement the kidneys. In addition, Epimedium supplements both yin and yang of the kidneys and harnesses ascendant liver yang. Phellodendron and Anemarrhena are two of the three assistants in this formula. They nourish kidney yin and drain fire. The third assistant, *Dang Gui* moistens and nourishes the blood and regulates the *chong* and *ren*.

Additions & subtractions:

For menopausal low back and knee soreness and weakness, add Ramus Loranthi Seu Visci (*Sang Ji Sheng*) and Cortex Eucommiae Ulmoidis (*Du Zhong*).

For menopausal insomnia with excessive dreams, add Semen Biotae Orientalis (*Bai Zi Ren*), Semen Zizyphi Spinosae (*Suan Zao Ren*), mix-fried Radix Glycyrrhizae (*Zhi Gan Cao*), Fructus Levis Tritici (*Fu Xiao Mai*), and Fructus Zizyphi Jujubae (*Da Zao*).

For menopausal night sweats, add Fructus Levis Tritici (*Fu Xiao Mai*), Concha Ostreae (*Mu Li*), and Radix Albus Paeoniae Lactiflorae (*Bai Shao*).

If night sweats are severe, add Fructus Levis Tritici (*Fu Xiao Mai*), Radix Ephedrae (*Ma Huang Gen*), and Radix Et Rhizoma Oryzae Sativae (*Nao Dao Gen Xu*).

For menopausal diarrhea caused by emotional upset in turn due to liver qi invading the spleen, add Radix Dioscoreae Oppositae (*Shan Yao*), Rhizoma Atractylodis Macrocephalae (*Bai Zhu*), Radix Saussureae Seu Vladimiriae (*Mu Xiang*), Fructus Zizyphi Jujubae (*Da Zao*), and mix-fried Radix Glycyrrhizae (*Zhi Gan Cao*). If this has gone on for some time, also add Fructus Terminaliae Chebulae (*He Zi*).

For menopausal fatigue, add Radix Astragali Membranacei (*Huang Qi*) and Radix Panacis Ginseng (*Ren Shen*).

For premenopausal early periods in women in their late 30s and early to mid 40s, add Radix Astragali Membranacei (*Huang Qi*), Radix Panacis Ginseng (*Ren Shen*), Radix Bupleuri (*Chai Hu*), Rhizoma Cimicifugae (*Sheng Ma*), and Gelatinum Corii Asini (*E Jiao*).

For perimenopausal breast distention, pain, and lumps, add Radix Scrophulariae Ningpoensis (*Xuan Shen*), Bulbus Fritillariae (*Bei Mu*), Concha Ostreae (*Mu Li*), Spica Prunellae Vulgaris (*Xia Gu Cao*), Herba Sargassii (*Hai Zao*), Thallus Algae (*Kun Bu*), and Semen Citri (*Ju He*).

For more prominent yin vacuity, subtract Curculigo and add Herba Ecliptae Prostratae (*Han Lian Cao*) and Fructus Ligustri Lucidi (*Nu Zhen Zi*).

For fluid dryness constipation, add Semen Cannabis Sativae (*Huo Ma Ren*), Herba Cistanchis (*Rou Cong Rong*), Radix Achyranthis Bidentatae (*Niu Xi*), Radix Polygoni Multiflori (*He Shou Wu*), and Fructus Immaturus Citri Seu Ponciri (*Zhi Shi*).

For yang vacuity, cold, damp pattern senile vaginitis, subtract Anemarrhena, Phellodendron, and Morinda and add Fructus Lycii Chinensis (*Gou Qi Zi*), Radix Dioscoreae Oppositae (*Shan Yao*), Radix Codonopsis Pilosulae (*Dang Shen*), Sclerotium Poriae Cocos (*Fu Ling*), and Fructus Rubi (*Fu Pen Zi*).

Comment: This is the single most effective TCM formula for the treatment of menopausal complaints. It can be made to treat almost every menopausal sign or symptom.

7

An Shen Ji
Spirit-quieting Formulas

Spirit-quieting formulas seek to treat emotional disturbances causing vexation and agitation, insomnia, excessive dreams, and palpitations. There are two basic types of spirit-quieting formulas. One subcategory is used for emotional disturbances due to vacuity and the other is used for emotional disturbances due to repletion. In the case of repletion, replete fire arising from the liver or stomach ascends to the heart where it disquiets the spirit. In the case of vacuity, blood and yin fail to nourish the spirit and thus it is not calm. Therefore, the subcategory of spirit-quieting formulas which mostly deals with repletion is called heavy, settling, spirit-quieting formulas. These formulas are mostly made from bitter, cold medicinals to drain fire and heavy, settling ingredients to press down ascendant yang. The subcategory of formulas which most deals with vacuity agitation and restlessness is called enriching and nourishing spirit-quieting formulas. These formulas mostly consist of blood-nourishing and yin-enriching medicinals assisted by vacuity heat clearing ingredients. However, because vacuity and repletion often go hand in hand in the kinds of counterflow inversion conditions associated with mental and emotional agitation, most formulas that quiet the spirit include a combination of heavy, settling ingredients, heat-clearing ingredients, and nourishing and supplementing ingredients.

7.1 *Zhong Zhen An Shen Ji* (Heavy, settling, spirit-quieting formulas)

Representative formula: *Zhu Sha An Shen Wan* (Cinnabar Quiet the Spirit Pills)

Composition:

Cinnabaris (*Zhu Sha*), 3g
Rhizoma Coptidis Chinensis (*huang Lian*), 6g
Radix Angelicae Sinensis (*Dang Gui*), 9g
raw Radix Rehmanniae (*Sheng Di*), 9g
Radix Glycyrrhizae (*Gan Cao*), 6g, mix-fried

Functions: Settles the heart and quiets the spirit, drains fire and nourishes yin

Indications: Hyperactivity of heart fire, yin and blood insufficiency. Neurosis, neurasthenia, mental depression, psychosis, anxiety attacks, insomnia, palpitations, and mitral valve prolapse

Main signs & symptoms: Heart vexation, spirit in chaos, insomnia, excessive dreams, severe palpitations, palpitations due to fright, possible sores on the tip of the tongue, if severe, a desire but inability to vomit, shortness of breath, forgetfulness, a red tongue, and a rapid, thready pulse

Contraindications:

1. Because of Cinnabar's toxicity, do not use in large doses or for prolonged periods of time. Do not use more than 2g per time and for more than 1 week.

Explanation of formula:

Within this formula, Cinnabar is the sovereign medicinal. It is heavy and settling and therefore quiets the heart spirit. Because it is cold, it is able to overwhelm heat. Thus it restrains floating fire. Coptis is bitter and cold and drains fire. It is the minister medicinal. It clears heat and eliminates vexation. Together, these two medicinals drain fire, clear heat, and eliminate vexation at the same time as heavily settling and quieting the spirit and will or orientation (*i.e.*, emotions). Thus they are the ruling ingredients in this formula. *Dang Gui* nourishes the blood. Raw Rehmannia enriches yin. Together they supplement yin and blood which have been consumed and damaged. Hence they are the assistant medicinals. Licorice regulates and harmonizes all these other medicinals. As a total combination, one part of this formula drains exuberant fire, while the other part supplements insufficient yin and blood. Heart fire is downborne below and yin and blood are filled up above.

Additions & subtractions:

If there is concomitant hot phlegm in the chest with chest oppression and possible nausea, add Semen Trichosanthis Kirlowii (*Gua Lou Ren*) and Caulis In Taeniis Bambusae (*Zhu Ru*).

If heart fire is more prominent and there is more pronounced insomnia and vexation and agitation, add Plumula Nelumbinis Nuciferae (*Lian Zi Xin*) and Fructus Gardeniae Jasminoidis (*Zhi Zi*).

Or specifically for insomnia, add Plumula Nelumbinis Nuciferae (*Lian Zi Xin*), Radix Polygalae Tenuifoliae (*Yuan Zhi*), and Sclerotium Pararadicis Poriae Cocos (*Fu Shen*).

If there is irritability with a sensation of heat in the chest, add Fructus Gardeniae Jasminoidis (*Shan Zhi Zi*) and Semen Praeparatum Sojae (*Dan Dou Chi*).

129

If the tip of the tongue is particularly red and dark or is ulcerated accompanied by reddish yellow, scanty urine, add Herba Lophatheri Gracilis (*Dan Zhu Ye*) and Medulla Junci Effusi (*Deng Xin Cao*).

Comment: The US FDA prohibits the internal prescription of Cinnabar.

7.2 *Zi Yang An Shen Ji* (Enriching & nourishing spirit-quieting formulas)

Representative formula: *Suan Zao Ren Tang* (Zizyphus Spinosa Decoction)

Composition:

Semen Zizyphi Spinosae (*Suan Zao Ren*), 18g
Radix Glycyrrhizae (*Gan Cao*), 3g
Rhizoma Anemarrhenae (*Zhi Mu*), 9g
Sclerotium Poriae Cocos (*Fu Ling*), 9g
Rhizoma Ligustici Wallichii (*Chuan Xiong*), 3g

Functions: Nourishes the blood and quiets the spirit, clears heat and eliminates vexation

Indications: Vacuity taxation, vacuity vexation, inability to sleep. Insomnia, nervous exhaustion, night sweats, poor memory, nightmares, rapid heart palpitations, crying and irritability in teething infants, neurasthenia, and schizophrenia

Main signs & symptoms: Heart palpitations, night sweats, dizziness and vertigo, dry throat and mouth, a red tongue, and a thready, rapid pulse

Formula explanation:

Zizyphus Spinosa nourishes liver blood and is the ruling medicinal for quieting the heart spirit. Its assistant is Ligusticum which regulates and nourishes liver blood. Poria tranquilizes the heart and quiets the spirit. Anemarrhena supplements insufficiency of yin at the same time as clearing internal flaring of fire. Thus it has the functions of enriching and clearing simultaneously, and Licorice clears heat and harmonizes the other medicinals.

Additions & subtractions:

For vacuous heart and gallbladder qi with waking frightened in the middle of the night, a pale tongue and fine, wiry pulse, add Radix Codonopsis Pilosulae (*Dang Shen*) and Os Draconis (*Long Gu*).

For night sweats, add Concha Ostreae (*Mu Li*) and Fructus Schizandrae Chinensis (*Wu Wei Zi*).

Also for night sweats, add Semen Biotae Orientalis (*Bai Zi Ren*) and Fructus Schizandrae Chinensis (*Wu Wei Zi*).

For severe vacuity fire, subtract Ligusticum and add Herba Ecliptae Prostratae (*Han Lian Cao*), Fructus Ligustri Lucidi (*Nu Zhen Zi*), and Radix Albus Paeoniae Lactiflorae (*Bai Shao*).

Also for severe yin vacuity with internal heat, add Radix Albus Paeoniae Lactiflorae (*Bai Shao*) and raw Radix Rehmanniae (*Sheng Di*).

For palpitations, add Dens Draconis (*Long Chi*) and Concha Ostreae (*Mu Li*).

For heart yin vacuity, add Tuber Ophiopogonis Japonicae (*Mai Dong*) and Semen Biotae Orientalis (*Bai Zi Ren*).

For heart blood vacuity, add Arillus Euphoriae Longanae (*Long Yan Rou*), Radix Salviae Miltiorrhizae (*Dan Shen*), Cortex Albizziae Julibrissinis (*He Huan Pi*), and Caulis Polygoni Multiflori (*Ye Jiao Teng*).

For heart qi vacuity, add Radix Codonopsis Pilosulae (*Dang Shen*) and Radix Pseudostellariae (*Tai Zi Shen*).

For heart yang vacuity, add Cortex Cinnamomi (*Rou Gui*) or Ramulus Cinnamomi (*Gui Zhi*).

Comment: Zizyphus Spinosa should be decocted before the other ingredients.

8

Kai Qiao Ji
Portal-opening Formulas

The formulas under this category are composed of ingredients which aromatically open the portals. These formulas are used in conditions when the spirit becomes confused and the portals become shut. Practically speaking, such conditions are associated with loss of consciousness and coma. In TCM, they are divided into replete and vacuity categories. Repletion patterns are blockage patterns. They are mostly due to gathering of exuberant evil qi which then block the portals of the heart. These blockages may be further subdivided into heat blockage and cold blockage. It is these repletion blockages which are the subject of this chapter.

Heat blockage is due to warm evils and heat toxins internally sinking into the pericardium. Cold blockage is due to cold evils and/or qi depression resulting in phlegm turbidity veiling the portals of the heart. In the first instance, the appropriate treatment principles are to clear heat and open the portals. In the second instance, the appropriate treatment principles are to warmly free the flow and open the portals.

The formulas in this category are primarily used in the form of patent medicines. This is because they are for emergency use and one cannot wait till a packet of herbs is made up and then decocted. It is also because some of the aromatic ingredients used do not lend themselves to decoction. These formulas also tend to be complicated in their composition.

Cautions & Contraindications:

1. Before employing formulas from this category, be sure the case is due to repletion. Do not use for atonic loss of consciousness.
2. If the case is due to *yang ming* division disease, use formulas from the draining and precipitating category.
3. Do not use these formulas for long-term administration since they are very scattering and dispersing and may easily damage the righteous.

8.1 *Liang Kai Ji* (Cool opening formulas)

Representative formula: *An Gong Niu Huang Wan* (Quieting the Palace Bezoar Pills)

Composition:

Calculus Bovis (*Niu Huang*), 30g
Tuber Curcumae (*Yu Jin*), 30g
Cornu Rhinocerotis (*Xi Jiao*), 30g
Rhizoma Coptidis Chinensis (*Huang Lian*), 30g
Radix Scutellariae Baicalensis (*Huang Qin*), 30g
Fructus Gardeniae Jasminoidis (*Zhi Zi*), 30g
Cinnabaris (*Zhu Sha*), 30g
Realgar (*Xiong Huang*), 30g
Secretio Moschi Moschiferi (*She Xiang*), 7.5g
Borneol (*Bing Pian*), 7.5g
Margarita (*Zhen Zhu*), 15g

Method of preparation & administration: Grind the above medicinals into fine powder and make into pills with honey weighing 3g apiece. Take 1 pill 2-3 times per day with warm water. Children should be given half the adult dose. If the patient is unconscious, the medicine may be administered by nasogastric tube.

Functions: Clears heat and opens the portals, sweeps away phlegm and resolves toxins

Indications: Warm and hot diseases, hot evils internally sinking into the pericardium, phlegm heat gathering and blocking the portals of the heart. Total or partial loss of consciousness due to acute encephalitis, acute meningitis, acute hepatitis, pneumonia, dysentery, uremia, hepatic coma, cerebrovascular accident, infantile convulsions, and schizophrenia

Main signs & symptoms: High fever, vexation and agitation, confused spirit, delirious speech, possible wind stroke with loss of consciousness and coma, infantile convulsions and spasms due to evil heat blocking internally

Contraindications:

1. Do not use during pregnancy.
2. Do not use in high doses or long-term due to the possibility of mercury toxicity from the Cinnabar.
3. Do not heat.

Formula explanation:

Within this formula, Bezoar clears heat and resolves toxins, sweeps away phlegm and opens the portals. Musk opens the portals and arouses the spirit. These are the sovereigns in this formula. There are several ministers in this formula. Rhinoceros Horn clears the heart, cools the blood, and resolves toxins. Coptis, Scutellaria, and Gardenia clear heat, drain fire, and resolve toxins. They help Bezoar clear fire from the pericardium. Borneol and Curcuma are aromatic. They free the portals and open blockage. Thus they help Musk open the portals and arouse the spirit. The assistants are Cinnabar, Pearl, and Realgar. Cinnabar and Pearl settles the heart and quiet the spirit, thus eliminating vexation, agitation, and disquiet. Realgar aids Bezoar in sweeping away phlegm and resolving toxins. Honey, which is used to bind the above ingredients into pills, is the messenger which harmonizes the stomach and regulates the center.

Additions & subtractions:

In cases with a vacuous, weak pulse, take with a decoction made from Radix Panacis Quinquefolii (*Xi Yang Shen*) to support the righteous.

In cases with a replete pulse, take with a decoction of Flos Lonicerae Japonicae (*Yin Hua*) and Herba Menthae (*Bo He*) to clear evil heat and penetrate the network vessels.

8.2 *Wen Kai Ji* (Warm opening formulas)

Representative formula: Su He Xiang Wan (Liquid Styrax Pills)

Composition:

Rhizoma Atractylodis Macrocephalae (*Bai Zhu*), 60g
Radix Saussureae Seu Vladimiriae (*Qing Mu Xiang*), 60g
Cornu Rhinocerotis (*Wu Xi Jiao*), 60g
Rhizoma Cyperi Rotundi (*Xiang Fu Zi*), 60g, stir-fried, remove the hairs
Cinnabaris (*Zhu Sha*), 60g, powdered, washed in water
Fructus Terminaliae Chebulae (*He Zi*), 60g, remove the skin
Lignum Santali Albi (*Bai Tan Xiang*), 60g
Lignum Aquilariae Agallochae (*Chen Xiang*), 60g
Benzoinum (*An Xi Xiang*), 60g, powdered
Secretio Moschi Moschiferi (*She Xiang*), 60g
Flos Caryophylli (*Ding Xiang*), 60g
Fructus Piperis Longi (*Bi Ba*), 60g
Borneol (*Long Nao*), 30g

Oleum Styracis Liquidis (*Su He Xiang You*), 30g
Gummum Olibani (*Ru Xiang*), 30g

Method of preparation & administration: Powder the above ingredients finely and use the Liquid Stryax Oil and white Honey to form pills. Take one 3g pill 1-2 times per day. The dose for children should be reduced based on the age and size of the child. If the patient is unconscious, this medicine can be introduced via a nasogastric tube.

Functions: Aromatically opens the portals, moves the qi and stops pain

Indications: Wind stroke, qi stroke, or cold stroke, *i.e.*, blockage and obstruction by cold evils, phlegm turbidity, or qi depression. Partial or total loss of consciousness due to cerebrovascular accident, uremia, or hepatic coma, encephalitis, hysteria, seizure disorders, psychosis, schizophrenia, postconcussion syndrome, dry sudden chaos (*i.e.*, cholera-like) disease, and angina pectoris, and coronary heart disease

Main signs & symptoms: Sudden collapse, loss of consciousness of human affairs, lock-jaw, possible strike of cold or qi blockage causing sudden heart and abdominal pain, if severe, confusion and inversion (*i.e.*, loss of consciousness), possible gathering of phlegm and qi obstruction, a pale, white face, cold breath issuing from the nose and mouth, cold hands and feet, a white, slimy tongue coating, and a deep, slow, forceful or wiry, tight, and forceful pulse

Contraindications:

1. Do not use during pregnancy.
2. Do not take in high doses or long-term for fear of mercury poisoning from the Cinnabar.
3. Do not heat.

Formula explanation:

In this formula, Styrax, Musk, Borneol, and Benzoinum aromatically open the portals and are the sovereign medicinals. They are aided by Saussurea, Sandalwood, Aquilaria, Frankincense, Cloves, and Cyperus as the ministers. These move the qi and resolve depression, scatter cold and transform turbidity. Thus they are able to resolve and eliminate depression and stagnation of the viscera and bowels, qi and blood. The assistant is Piper Longum, which when combined with the above 10 types of aromatic medicinals, helps strengthen the scattering of cold, the stopping of pain, and the opening of depression. They are also aided by Rhinoceros Horn which resolves toxins and Cinnabar which settles the heart and quiets the spirit. Atractylodis supplements the qi and fortifies the spleen, dries dampness and transforms turbidity. Terminalia astringes and restrains the qi. When combined with all these aromatic medicinals, it is able to supplement the qi and restrain it, thus preventing those acrid, aromatic ingredients from consuming and scattering the righteous qi.

9

Gu Se Ji
Securing & Astringing Formulas

One of the five functions of the qi is to restrain blood, essence, and fluids within the body. Formulas within the securing and astringing category are meant to control the unwanted loss or discharge of blood, essence, or body fluids to the outside of the body. Typically, such formulas are made up of a combination of qi-supplementing medicinals with astringent ingredients, since loss of securing is ascribed to vacuity and insufficiency of the lungs, spleen, and/or kidneys. There are four main subcategories of securing and astringing formulas: 1) formulas which secure the exterior and stop sweating, 2) formulas which astringe the intestines and stem desertion (*i.e.*, prolonged diarrhea or dysentery), 3) formulas which astringe the essence and stop loss (semen), and 4) formulas which secure flooding (*i.e.*, uterine bleeding) and stop abnormal vaginal discharge. Although the lungs, spleen, and kidneys all share in the control of qi, the kidneys especially control opening and closing in general and closing of the treasuries in particular. Thus most of the formulas in this category contain kidney-supplementing medicinals.

Cautions & Contraindications:

1. Do not use in cases of loss, discharge, and emission due to repletion.
2. Do not use if there are retained or hidden evils.

3. In the treatment of diseases characterized by unwanted loss of blood, essence, and body fluids due to vacuity of righteous qi, it is necessary to treat both the root and branch simultaneously.

9.1 *Gu Biao Zhi Han Ji* (Exterior-securing, perspiration-stopping formulas)

Representative formula: *Mu Li San* (Oyster Shell Powder)

Composition:

Radix Astragali Membranacei (*Huang Qi*), 15g
Radix Ephedrae (*Ma Huang Gen*), 9g
Concha Ostreae (*Mu Li*), 15-30g
Fructus Levis Tritici (*Fu Xiao Mai*), 15-30g

Functions: Secures the exterior and restrains the sweat

Indications: All types of vacuity and insufficiency accompanied by spontaneous perspiration

Main signs & symptoms: Spontaneous sweating on slight or no movement, prolonged or excessive sweating which will not stop, palpitations, shortness of breath, vexation, fatigue, a pale red tongue, and a fine, weak pulse

Contraindications:

1. Do not use unmodified to treat night sweating due to yin vacuity, flaring fire.
2. Do not use unmodified to treat profuse, oily sweating with cold limbs and a weak pulse due to yang collapse.

Formula explanation:

Within this formula, Oyster Shell is the sovereign medicinal. It boosts yin and subdues yang, thus simultaneously eliminating vexation and restraining perspiration. Astragalus boosts the qi and replenishes the defensive, secures the exterior and stops sweating. It is the minister medicinal. Radix Ephedrae in particular stops sweating, while Fructus Levis Tritici boosts heart qi, nourishes heart blood, clears the heart and eliminated vexation, and stops the discharge of sweat. These two are the assistant medicinals. When combined together, these medicinals nourish yin, secure the muscles and exterior, clear heat from the heart, and stop sweating.

Additions & subtractions:

For more pronounced defensive qi vacuity, add Fructus Schizandrae Chinensis (*Wu Wei Zi*).

For spleen qi vacuity, add Radix Codonopsis Pilosulae (*Dang Shen*) and Rhizoma Atractylodis Macrocephalae (*Bai Zhu*).

For yang vacuity, add Rhizoma Atractylodis Macrocephalae (*Bai Zhu*) and Radix Praeparatus Aconiti Carmichaeli (*Fu Zi*).

For blood vacuity, add Radix Polygoni Multiflori (*He Shou Wu*) and prepared Radix Rehmanniae (*Shu Di*).

Also for blood vacuity, add prepared Radix Rehmanniae (*Shu Di*) and Gelatinum Corii Asini (*E Jiao*).

For yin vacuity with night sweats, add prepared Radix Rehmanniae (*Shu Di*), Semen Biotae Orientalis (*Bai Zi Ren*), and Radix Albus Paeoniae Lactiflorae (*Bai Shao*).

For insomnia, add Semen Biotae Orientalis (*Bai Zi Ren*) and Semen Zizyphi Spinosae (*Suan Zao Ren*).

9.2 *Se Chang Gu Tuo Ji* (Intestine-astringing, desertion-stemming formulas)

Representative formulas:

A. *Zhen Ren Yang Zang Tang* (True Man Nourish the Viscera Decoction)

Composition:

Radix Panacis Ginseng (*Ren Shen*), 6g
Radix Angelicae Sinensis (*Dang Gui*), 9g
Rhizoma Atractylodis Macrocephalae (*Bai Zhu*), 12g
Semen Myristicae Fragrantis (*Rou Dou Kou*), 12g, dry roasted
Cortex Cinnamomi (*Rou Gui*), 3g
Radix Glycyrrhizae (*Gan Cao*), 6g, mix-fried
Radix Albus Paeoniae Lactiflorae (*Bai Shao*), 15g
Radix Saussureae Seu Vladimiriae (*Mu Xiang*), 9g
Fructus Terminaliae Chebulae (*He Zi*), 12g
Pericarpium Papaveris Sominiferae (*Ying Su Ke*), 20g, honey mix-fried

Functions: Astringes the intestines and stems desertion, warms and supplements the spleen and kidneys

Indications: Spleen/kidney vacuity cold, prolonged diarrhea and dysentery. Chronic colitis, chronic diarrhea in children, Crohn's disease, ulcerative colitis, chronic dysentery, celiac syndrome, and pancreatic dysfunction

Main signs & symptoms: Slippery desertion diarrhea, abdominal pain which likes both pressure and warmth, red and white dysentery, bloody stools, tenesmus, fatigue, diminished appetite, soreness and weakness of the low back and knees, a pale tongue with a thin, white coating, and a slow, thready pulse

Contraindications:

1. Do not use in the beginning stages of diarrhea and dysentery.
2. Do not use in repletion, stagnation, or damp heat patterns.
3. Do not eat or drink alcohol, wheat, cold, raw foods, fish, or greasy, fatty foods.

Formula explanation:

Within this formula, Cinnamon is the sovereign medicinal. It warms the kidneys and spleen. Nutmeg likewise warms the kidneys and spleen but it also astringes the intestines. Terminalia astringes the intestines and stops diarrhea. Ginseng and Atractylodis boost the qi and fortify the spleen. These are the minister medicinals which assist the sovereign medicinal in warming the kidneys and spleen.

Additions & subtractions:

For rectal prolapse, add Radix Astragali Membranacei (*Huang Qi*) and Rhizoma Cimicifugae (*Sheng Ma*).

For diarrhea with undigested food in the stools and chilled extremities, add Radix Praeparatus Aconiti Carmichaeli (*Fu Zi*) and dry Rhizoma Zingiberis (*Gan Jiang*).

For tenesmus, add Semen Arecae Catechu (*Bing Lang*).

For cold limbs and a deep, weak pulse due to severe vacuity cold of the spleen and kidneys, subtract Licorice and add either dry Rhizoma

Zingiberis (*Gan Jiang*) or Radix Praeparatus Aconiti Carmichaeli (*Fu Zi*) to warm the spleen and kidneys.

B. *Si Shen Wan* (Four Spirits Pills)

Composition:

Semen Myristicae Fragrantis (*Rou Dou Kou*), 9g
Fructus Psoraleae Corylifoliae (*Bu Gu Zhi*), 12g
Fructus Schizandrae Chinensis (*Wu Wei Zi*), 9g
Fructus Evodiae Rutecarpae (*Wu Zhu Yu*), 6g
raw Rhizoma Zingiberis (*Sheng Jiang*), 3g
Fructus Zizyphi Jujubae (*Da Zao*), 5 pieces

Functions: Warms and supplements the kidneys, astringes the intestines and stops diarrhea

Indications: Spleen/kidney vacuity cold. Chronic colitis, chronic dysentery, autonomic dystonia of the intestinal tract, intestinal tuberculosis, allergic colitis, tabes dorsalis, and pancreatic dysfunction

Main signs & symptoms: Fifth watch diarrhea (*i.e.*, cockcrow diarrhea), no thought for food or drink, prolonged diarrhea which will not heal, abdominal pain, low back soreness, chilled extremities, exhausted spirit, lack of strength, a pale tongue, and a deep, slow, forceless pulse

Contraindications:

1. Do not use unmodified if there is stagnation or accumulation within the stomach and intestines.

Formula explanation:

In this formula, Psoralea is acrid and bitter and its nature is hot. It supplements the *ming men* and therefore is an essential medicinal for strengthening fire and boosting earth. It is the sovereign medicinal within this formula. Nutmeg warms the spleen and kidneys, astringes the intestines, and stops diarrhea. Evodia also warms the spleen and kidneys as well as scatters cold and eliminates dampness. These are the minister medicinals. Schizandra is a warming and astringing ingredient. Fresh Ginger scatters cold and moves water. Red Dates enrich and nourish the spleen and stomach. These are the assistant medicinals. Taken as a whole, this formula warms the spleen and kidneys, astringes the large intestine, and augments transportation and transformation. When these are accomplished, diarrhea automatically stops and the disease is completely cured.

Additions & subtractions:

For rectal prolapse, add Radix Astragali Membranacei (*Huang Qi*) and Rhizoma Cimicifugae (*Sheng Ma*).

Also for rectal prolapse, add Radix Astragali Membranacei (*Huang Qi*) and Rhizoma Atractylodis Macrocephalae (*Bai Zhu*).

For cold hands and feet, add Radix Praeparatus Aconiti Carmichaeli (*Fu Zi*) and Cortex Cinnamomi (*Rou Gui*).

For lower abdominal pain, subtract Evodia and Schizandra and add Radix Saussureae Seu Vladimiriae (*Mu Xiang*) and Fructus Foeniculi Vulgaris (*Xiao Hui Xiang*).

For interior cold with abdominal pain and nausea, add *Li Zhong Wan* (Rectify the Center Pills), *i.e.*, Radix Panacis Ginseng (*Ren Shen*), Rhizoma Atractylodis Macrocephalae (*Bai Zhu*), mix-fried Radix

Glycyrrhizae (*Zhi Gan Cao*), and dry Rhizoma Zingiberis (*Gan Jiang*).

Comment: The previous formula is for more pronounced spleen vacuity with relatively less kidney yang vacuity. This formula is for more pronounced kidney vacuity and less obvious spleen vacuity.

9.3 *Se Jing Zhi Wei Ji* (Essence-astringing, loss-stopping formulas)

Representative formula: *Sang Piao Xiao San* (Ootheca Mantidis Powder)

Composition:

Ootheca Mantidis (*Sang Piao Xiao*), 12g
Radix Polygalae Tenuifoliae (*Yuan Zhi*), 6g
Rhizoma Acori Graminei (*Chang Pu*), 9g
Os Draconis (*Long Gu*), 18g
Radix Panacis Ginseng (*Ren Shen*), 9g
Sclerotium Pararadicis Poriae Cocos (*Fu Shen*), 9g
Radix Angelicae Sinensis (*Dang Gui*), 9g
Plastrum Testudinis (*Gui Ban*), 15g, vinegar mix-fried

Functions: Regulates and supplements the heart and kidneys, astringes the essence and stops loss

Indications: Heart/kidney dual vacuity. Polyuria, spermatorrhea, nocturnal emission, turbid urine due to cystitis, loss of memory due to nervous exhaustion, chronic nephritis, diabetes mellitus, diabetes insipidus, tubular acidosis, primary aldosteronism, hyperparathyroidism, neurosis, prolapsed uterus, and autonomic dystonia

Main signs & symptoms: Frequent urination possibly the color of rice-washing water, absentmindedness, forgetfulness, diminished appetite, if severe, incontinence and seminal emission, a pale tongue with thin, white coating, and a deep and weak or slow, fine, and weak pulse

Contraindications:

1. Do not use for incontinence for exuberant heat in the lower burner.
2. Do not use for damp heat in the lower burner.

Formula explanation:

Within this formula, Mantis Egg Cases supplement the kidneys and boost the essence, secure the floating and stop loss. Thus they are the sovereign medicinal in this formula. Dragon Bone restrains the heart spirit and astringes essence qi. Plastrum Testudinis boosts yin qi and supplements the heart and kidneys. These are the minister medicinals. Ginseng supplements the central qi, while *Dang Gui* nourishes heart blood. Spirit of Poria quiets the heart spirit. These are the assistant medicinals. Polygala and Acorus quiet the spirit and tranquilize the will or orientation (*i.e.*, emotions). They also connect and free the flow between the heart and kidneys. These are simultaneously assistant and messenger medicinals. As a whole, this formula is able to supplement the kidneys and boost the essence, astringe the essence and stop loss. It is also able to supplement the heart and nourish the spirit, connecting the kidneys and heart above and below.

Additions & subtractions:

For spermatorrhea, add Fructus Corni Officinalis (*Shan Zhu Yu*) and Semen Astragali Complanati (*Sha Yuan Ji Li*).

Also for spermatorrhea with fine, weak pulse, subtract Polygala and add Fructus Rosae Laevigatae (*Jin Ying Zi*) and Fructus Schizandrae Chinensis (*Wu Wei Zi*).

147

For enuresis, add Fructus Rubi (*Fu Pen Zi*) and Fructus Alpiniae Oxyphyllae (*Yi Zhi Ren*).

For dribbling urination in the elderly, subtract Polygala and add Radix Astragali Membranacei (*Huang Qi*) and Fructus Corni Officinalis (*Shan Zhu Yu*).

For neurasthenia with insomnia, forgetfulness, and palpitations, add Fructus Schizandrae Chinensis (*Wu Wei Zi*) and Semen Zizyphi Spinosae (*Suan Zao Ren*).

For diabetic polyuria, add Radix Dioscoreae Oppositae (*Shan Yao*) and Fructus Corni Officinalis (*Shan Zhu Yu*).

For severe kidney yang vacuity with chill, add Radix Morindae (*Ba Ji Tian*), Cortex Cinnamomi (*Rou Gui*), and Radix Praeparatus Aconiti Carmichaeli (*Fu Zi*).

For unstoppable incontinence, add *Suo Quan Wan* (Lock the Spring Pills), *i.e.*, Fructus Alpiniae Oxyphyllae (*Yi Zhi Ren*), Radix Linderae Strychnifoliae (*Wu Yao*), and Radix Dioscoreae Oppositae (*Shan Yao*).

Comment: This formula is primarily for enuresis and polyuria and only secondarily for spermatorrhea for which it needs to be modified as above.

9.4 *Gu Beng Zhi Dai Ji* (Securing flooding, stopping vaginal discharge formulas)

Representative formulas:

A. *Gu Chong Tang* (Secure the *Chong* Decoction)

Composition:

Radix Astragali Membranacei (*Huang Qi*), 30g

Rhizoma Atractylodis Macrocephalae (*Bai Zhu*), 18g, stir-fried
Fructus Corni Officinalis (*Shan Zhu Yu*), 24g
Radix Albus Paeoniae Lactiflorae (*Bai Shao*), 12g
calcined Concha Ostreae (*Duan Mu Li*), 24g
calcined Os Draconis (*Duan Long Gu*), 24g
Os Sepiae Seu Sepiellae (*Hai Piao Xiao*), 12g
Galla Rhi Chinensis (*Wu Bei Zi*), 1.5g
carbonized Fibra Stipulae Trachycarpi (*Zong Lu Tan*), 6g
Radix Rubiae Cordifoliae (*Qian Cao*), 9g

Method of preparation & administration: Precook the two calcined ingredients before adding the other medicinals to the decoction. Grind the Galla Rhi Chinensis into a fine powder, divide into 2 portions, and take 1 portion with the strained decoction, 2 times per day.

Functions: Boosts the qi and fortifies the spleen, secures the *chong* and stops bleeding

Indications: Uterine bleeding due to spleen/stomach vacuity weakness, qi and blood vacuity, and lack of securing of the *chong*. Functional uterine bleeding, excessive lochiorrhea, and bleeding peptic ulcers

Main signs & symptoms: Excessive uterine bleeding which is pale in color and thin in consistency, palpitations, shortness of breath, a pale tongue, and a large, vacuous or fine, weak pulse

Contraindications:

1. Do not use if hemorrhaging is so severe there are symptoms of yang collapse, such as perspiration, cold extremities, and a minute, hard-to-find pulse. In that case, use *Du Shen Tang* (Solitary Ginseng Decoction) until the condition has stabilized.

Formula explanation:

In this formula, Astragalus and Atractylodis are the sovereign medicinals. They boost the qi and fortify the spleen, restrain the blood and secure the *chong*. The minister medicinals are Cornus and White Peony. They enrich yin and nourish the blood as well as astringe the liver and kidneys respectively. Thus they help in securing the *chong mai*. The assistants consist of Dragon Bone, Oyster Shell, Cuttlefish Bone, Schizandra, and carbonized Trachycarpus. These ingredients astringe essence and stop bleeding. It should be remembered that, according to TCM theory, menstrual blood is the manifestation of essence in women. Rubia is the messenger. It quickens the blood and stops bleeding. It is, therefore, able to prevent blood stasis due to the heavy use of these other securing and astringing medicinals.

Additions & subtractions:

If complicated by yang vacuity as manifest by listlessness, a pale facial color, chilled extremities, and a weak pulse, add Radix Panacis Ginseng (*Ren Shen*) and Radix Praeparatus Aconiti Carmichaeli (*Fu Zi*).

If complicated by an element of heat, add raw Radix Rehmanniae (*Sheng Di*).

If due to a fit of anger, add Radix Bupleuri (*Chai Hu*).

If the condition does not improve after two days of the above treatment, subtract Trachycarpus and add Gelatinum Corii Asini (*E Jiao*).

For melena due to spleen qi vacuity, subtract Dragon Bone, Oyster Shell, and Galla Rhi Chinensis and add Radix Dioscoreae Oppositae (*Shan Yao*) to nourish spleen yin.

B. *Wan Dai Tang* (Finish Abnormal Vaginal Discharge Decoction)

Composition:

Rhizoma Atractylodis Macrocephalae (*Bai Zhu*), 30g, earth stir-fried
Radix Dioscoreae Oppositae (*Shan Yao*), 30g
Radix Panacis Ginseng (*Ren Shen*), 6g
Radix Albus Paeoniae Lactiflorae (*Bai Shao*), 15g, wine stir-fried
Semen Plantaginis (*Che Qian Zi*), 9g, wine stir-fried
Rhizoma Atractylodis (*Cang Zhu*), 9g, processed
Radix Glycyrrhizae (*Gan Cao*), 3g
Pericarpium Citri Reticulatae (*Chen Pi*), 1.5g
blackened Herba Seu Flos Schizonepetae Tenuifoliae (*Hei Jing Jie*),
    1.5g
Radix Bupleuri (*Chai Hu*), 1.8g

Functions: Supplements the center and fortifies the spleen, transforms dampness and stops vaginal discharge

Indications: Spleen vacuity/liver depression, damp turbidity pouring downward. Abnormal vaginal discharge, hemophilus vaginitis, vulvitis, cervical inflammation, diarrhea, edema during pregnancy, edema during menstruation, and headache

Main signs & symptoms: Abnormal vaginal discharge which is colored white or pale yellow and is clear, thin, and without odor, an ashen, white facial color, fatigue, loose stools, a pale tongue with white coating, and a relaxed/retarded or soggy, weak pulse

Contraindications:

1. Do not use if the vaginal discharge is thick, dark yellow, contains blood, or is foul smelling and the patient has a yellow tongue coating and a wiry pulse.

Formula explanation:

In this formula, Ginseng, Atractylodis, and Dioscorea are the sovereign medicinals. They are all qi-supplementing, spleen-fortifying ingredients. Atractylodis is additionally able to dry dampness. Dioscorea simultaneously astringes the essence. Thus this combination helps to fortify the spleen and stop abnormal vaginal discharge. Atractylodis and Orange Peel dry dampness and transport the spleen. They aromatically move the qi. They enable the sovereign ingredients to supplement without causing stagnation. Plantago blandly percolates and disinhibits dampness. It helps remove water dampness via urination. These all are the minister medicinals. This combination of sovereign and minister medicinals stops abnormal vaginal discharge without retaining dampness and disinhibits dampness without damaging the righteous. White Peony soothes the liver and supports the spleen. Bupleurum upbears yang. They assist in assuring that damp qi is not flow downward into the interior. Schizonepeta enters the blood division, expels wind, overwhelms dampness, and thus stops vaginal discharge. These are the assistant medicinals. Licorice regulates these medicinals and harmonizes the center. Therefore, it is the messenger medicinal in this formula.

Additions & subtractions:

For soreness and pain of the low back, add Cortex Eucommiae Ulmoidis (*Du Zhong*), Semen Cuscutae (*Tu Si Zi*), and Radix Dipsaci (*Xu Duan*).

Also for soreness and pain in the low back, add Ramus Loranthi Seu Visci (*Sang Ji Sheng*), Cortex Eucommiae Ulmoidis (*Du Zhong*), and Rhizoma Cibotii Barometsis (*Gou Ji*).

For cold abdominal pain, add Folium Artemisiae Argyii (*Ai Ye*), Rhizoma Cyperi Rotundi (*Xiang Fu*), and Radix Linderae Strychnifoliae (*Wu Yao*).

Also for cold abdominal pain, add Radix Linderae Strychnifoliae (*Wu Yao*), Fructus Foeniculi Vulgaris (*Xiao Hui Xiang*), and blast-fried Rhizoma Zingiberis (*Pao Jiang*).

For lower abdominal and hypochondrial pain, add Rhizoma Corydalis Yanhusuo (*Yan Hu*) and Rhizoma Cyperi Rotundi (*Xiang Fu*).

For prolonged vacuity and chill with a very thin discharge, add Cornu Degelatinum Cervi (*Lu Jiao Shuang*), Cortex Cinnamomi (*Rou Gui*), Radix Morindae (*Ba Ji Tian*), and Os Sepiae Seu Sepiellae (*Wu Zei Gu*).

To strengthen the securing and astringing effect of this formula, add calcined Os Draconis (*Duan Long Gu*) and calcined Concha Ostreae (*Duan Mu Li*).

逍遥散用当归芍
柴苓术草加姜薄
散郁除蒸功最奇
调经八味丹栀着

Mnemonic verse for learning *Xiao Yao San*

10

Li Qi Ji
Qi-rectifying Formulas

Qi-rectifying formulas address either of two anomalies of the qi. In the first case, there may be qi stagnation. This means the qi does not move freely as it should. Usually this is due to the liver losing its control over coursing and discharge. However, because the qi transports and transforms the blood, dampness, phlegm, and food, qi stagnation may be complicated by depression of any of these yin substances. In addition, if qi becomes depressed, it may transform into depressive heat or fire. Therefore, the subcategory of qi-rectifying formulas known as qi-moving formulas commonly include medicinals which treat one or more of these complicating depressions. This subcategory is itself divided into two groups of formulas: 1) those formulas which treat stagnation of the spleen and stomach qi with upper abdominal distention, belching, nausea, and possible vomiting and 2) those formulas which treat liver depression, qi stagnation with distention and pain in the lateral costal region with possible distention and pain more prominent in the lower abdomen.

Secondly, if qi accumulates, because it is yang, it will eventually counterflow upward. This may affect the downward flow of the qi of the stomach and lungs. In such cases, the qi of this viscus and bowel may counterflow upward. Therefore, the second subcategory of qi-rectifying formulas is known as qi-downbearing formulas. These formulas downbear upwardly counterflowing qi, thus insuring the regular and harmonious arising of clear yang and the downbearing of turbid yin.

Qi-rectifying ingredients have many similarities to exterior-resolving medicinals. Both groups can be referred to as windy medicinals. This is because both groups tend to be acrid, drying, ascending, and out-thrusting. Even within the downbearing group of qi-rectifying formulas, downbearing medicinals are usually used in tandem with dry, acrid medicinals to upbear yang and thrust outward. Due to their dry, windy nature, qi-rectifying ingredients can consume yin and blood if improperly used and damage the righteous qi.

Cautions & Contraindications:

1. Use with care in patients with blood vacuity, yin vacuity, or insufficient body fluids.
2. Do not use indefinitely once the condition improves.

10.1 *Xing Qi Ji* (Moving qi formulas)

Representative formulas:

A. *Yue Ju Wan* (Escape Restraint Pills)

Composition:

Rhizoma Cyperi Rotundi (*Xiang Fu*), 12g
Rhizoma Atractylodis (*Cang Zhu*), 12g
Rhizoma Ligustici Wallichii (*Chuan Xiong*), 12g
Fructus Gardeniae Jasminoidis (*Zhi Zi*), 12g
Massa Medica Fermentata (*Shen Qu*), 12g

Functions: Moves the qi and resolves depression

Indications: Qi depression with chest and diaphragm glomus and oppression. Gastrointestinal neurosis, gastric or duodenal ulcer, chronic gastritis, infectious hepatitis, chronic cholecystitis, cholelithiasis, intercostal neuralgia, irregular menstruation, and dysmenorrhea

Main signs & symptoms: Epigastric and abdominal distention and pain, belching, burping, acid eructations, nausea, vomiting, indigestion, a thin, white or slimy, glossy tongue coating, and a wiry or wiry, slippery pulse

Contraindications:

1. Do not use unmodified for stagnation due to vacuity.

Formula explanation:

Because qi depression may cause depression of blood, phlegm, fire, dampness, and/or food, each ingredient in this formula addresses one of these depressions. Cyperus is the main ingredient in this formula. It moves the qi and resolves depression, thus treating qi depression. Ligusticum quickens the blood and dispels stasis, thus treating blood depression. Gardenia clears heat and drains fire, thus treating fire depression. Atractylodis dries dampness and transports the spleen, thus treating damp depression. Massa Medica Fermentata disperses food and conducts stagnation, thus treating food depression. Qi depression leads to gathering of dampness and the generation of phlegm. If the qi dynamic flows smoothly, these five depressions are resolved and the resolution of phlegm depression follows suit. Therefore, it is generally not necessary to add any medicinals specifically for it.

Additions & subtractions:

For more serious qi depression, add Radix Saussureae Seu Vladimiriae (*Mu Xiang*) and Fructus Citri Seu Ponciri (*Zhi Ke*).

For even more serious qi depression, to the above add Pericarpium Citri Reticulatae (*Chen Pi*) and Pericarpium Viridis Citri Reticulatae (*Qing Pi*).

Also for more serious qi depression, add Radix Saussureae Seu Vladimiriae (*Mu Xiang*) and Tuber Curcumae (*Yu Jin*).

For lancinating pain in the chest and lateral costal regions, add Tuber Curcumae (*Yu Jin*) and Flos Carthami Tinctorii (*Hong Hua*).

For more serious blood depression, add Semen Pruni Persicae (*Tao Ren*) and Flos Carthami Tinctorii (*Hong Hua*).

For even more serious blood depression, to the above add Radix Salviae Miltiorrhizae (*Dan Shen*) and Radix Angelicae Sinensis (*Dang Gui*).

For more serious damp depression, add Sclerotium Poriae Cocos (*Fu Ling*) and Rhizoma Alismatis (*Ze Xie*).

For even more serious damp depression, to the above add Semen Plantaginis (*Che Qian Zi*) and Semen Coicis Lachryma-jobi (*Yi Yi Ren*).

For flatulence due to damp depression, add Sclerotium Poriae Cocos (*Fu Ling*) and Ramulus Cinnamomi (*Gui Zhi*) to move the qi and transform dampness.

For more serious food stagnation, add Fructus Germinatus Hordei Vulgaris (*Mai Ya*) and Fructus Crataegi (*Shan Zha*).

For loss of appetite, nausea, and vomiting due to food stagnation, add Fructus Germinatus Hordei Vulgaris (*Mai Ya*) and Caulis Perillae Frutescentis (*Su Gen*).

For even more serious food depression, to the above add Endothelium Corneum Gigeriae Galli (*Ji Nei Jin*) and Semen Arecae Catechu (*Bing Lang*).

For severe bloating and distention, add Pericarpium Viridis Citri Reticulatae (*Qing Pi*), Pericarpium Citri Reticulatae (*Chen Pi*), Fructus Immaturus Citri Seu Ponciri (*Zhi Shi*), and Semen Arecae Catechu (*Bing Lang*).

For more serious phlegm depression, add Rhizoma Pinelliae Ternatae (*Ban Xia*) and Rhizoma Arisaematis (*Tian Nan Xing*).

Also for more serious phlegm depression, add Rhizoma Pinelliae Ternatae (*Ban Xia*) and Pericarpium Citri Reticulatae (*Chen Pi*) to rectify the qi and transform phlegm.

For even more serious phlegm depression, add Pericarpium Citri Reticulatae (*Chen Pi*), Rhizoma Pinelliae Ternatae (*Ban Xia*), either Pericarpium Trichosanthis Kirlowii (*Gua Lou Pi*), Fructus Trichosanthis Kirlowii (*Gua Lou*), or Semen Trichosanthis Kirlowii (*Gua Lou Ren*), and bile-processed Rhizoma Arisaematis (*Dan Nan Xing*).

If liver fire predominates, subtract Atractylodis and add Radix Albus Paeoniae Lactiflorae (*Bai Shao*) and Cortex Radicis Moutan (*Dan Pi*).

For more serious fire depression, add Rhizoma Coptidis Chinensis (*Huang Lian*) and Radix Scutellariae Baicalensis (*Huang Qin*).

For lateral costal and hypochondrial pain with acid eructation, add Rhizoma Coptidis Chinensis (*Huang Lian*) and Fructus Evodiae Rutecarpae (*Wu Zhu Yu*).

For dysmenorrhea or mental depression, add Tuber Curcumae (*Yu Jin*) and Fructus Citri Sacrodactylis (*Fo Shou*).

159

Also for dysmenorrhea, add Tuber Curcumae (*Yu Jin*), Herba Leonuri Heterophylli (*Yi Mu Cao*), Radix Angelicae Sinensis (*Dang Gui*), and Radix Albus Paeoniae Lactiflorae (*Bai Shao*).

For heat and stasis in the liver with hypochondrial pain, a yellow tongue coating, and a wiry, rapid pulse, add Rhizoma Corydalis Yanhusuo (*Yan Hu*).

For abdominal pain due to cold stagnation, add Rhizoma Alpiniae Officinari (*Gao Liang Jiang*).

For even more serious abdominal pain due to cold stagnation, to the above add Fructus Evodiae Rutecarpae (*Wu Zhu Yu*) and dry Rhizoma Zingiberis (*Gan Jiang*) and subtract Gardenia.

Comment: Depression in this context does not mean emotional depression as understood in the West. Here it is used as a technical term within TCM.

B. *Ban Xia Hou Po Tang* (Pinellia & Magnolia Decoction)

Composition:

Rhizoma Pinelliae Ternatae (*Ban Xia*), 12g
Cortex Magnoliae Officinalis (*Hou Po*), 9g
Sclerotium Poriae Cocos (*Fu Ling*), 12g
raw Rhizoma Zingiberis (*Sheng Jiang*), 9g
Folium Perillae Frutescentis (*Su Ye*), 6g

Functions: Moves the qi and scatters nodulation, downbears counterflow and transforms phlegm

Indications: Plum pit qi. Neurotic esophageal stenosis, globus hystericus, gastrointestinal neurosis, chronic laryngitis, tracheitis, neurasthenia, morning sickness, bronchitis, hysteria, neurosis, recurrent palpitations, asthma, pertussis, toxemia during pregnancy, and edema

Main signs & symptoms: The sensation of something stuck in the throat which cannot be spit up or swallowed down, chest and lateral costal fullness and oppression, possible cough with copious phlegm, possible vomiting, a white, moist or slimy, glossy tongue coating, and a wiry or wiry, slippery pulse

Contraindications:

1. Do not use in patients with a flushed face, bitter taste in the mouth, and a red tongue with scant coating. This means those with yin vacuity or heat due to liver depression, stagnant qi transforming into internal heat.

Formula explanation:

This formula uses Pinellia to transform phlegm and scatter nodulation, downbear counterflow and harmonize the stomach. It is the sovereign medicinal in this prescription. Magnolia lowers the qi and eliminates fullness. It assists Pinellia in scattering nodulation and downbearing counterflow. Poria, sweet and bland, percolates dampness. It assists Pinellia in transforming phlegm. Magnolia and Poria are this formula's minister medicinals. Fresh Ginger, acrid and warm, scatters nodulation, harmonizes the stomach, and stops vomiting, while Folium Perillae aromatically moves the qi, rectifies the lungs, and soothes the liver. These are the assistant and messenger medicinals.

Additions & subtractions:

For concomitant qi vacuity, add *Si Mo San* (Four Ground [Ingredients] Powder), *i.e.*, Radix Panacis Ginseng (*Ren Shen*), Semen Arecae Catechu (*Bing Lang*), Lignum Aquilariae Agallochae (*Chen Xiang*), and Radix Linderae Strychnifoliae (*Wu Yao*).

161

For severe qi stagnation, add Radix Bupleuri (*Chai Hu*), Tuber Curcumae (*Yu Jin*), Rhizoma Cyperi Rotundi (*Xiang Fu*), and Pericarpium Viridis Citri Reticulatae (*Qing Pi*).

Also for severe qi stagnation, add *Xiao Yao San* (Rambling Powder), *i.e.*, Radix Bupleuri (*Chai Hu*), Radix Angelicae Sinensis (*Dang Gui*), Radix Albus Paeoniae Lactiflorae (*Bai Shao*), Rhizoma Atractylodis Macrocephalae (*Bai Zhu*), Sclerotium Poriae Cocos (*Fu Ling*), mixfried Radix Glycyrrhizae (*Zhi Gan Cao*), and Herba Menthae (*Bo He*).

For blockage and obstruction to swallowing with glomus and fullness of the chest and diaphragm, a slimy, white tongue coating, and a wiry, slippery pulse, add Tuber Curcumae (*Yu Jin*) and Fructus Amomi (*Sha Ren*).

For vomiting of phlegmy substances but no thirst, subtract Magnolia, Perilla, and Poria. This results in *Xiao Ban Xia Tang* (Minor Pinellia Decoction).

Also for vomiting, add Fructus Amomi (*Sha Ren*), Flos Caryophylli (*Ding Xiang*), and Fructus Cardamomi (*Bai Dou Kou*).

If there is a red tongue with a scant, dry coating, add Radix Glehniae Littoralis (*Sha Shen*), Tuber Ophiopogonis Japonicae (*Mai Dong*), and Radix Scrophulariae Ningpoensis (*Xuan Shen*).

Also, to help protect stomach fluids from these warm, acrid, drying medicinals or to treat a milder condition with less phlegm dampness, one can add Fructus Zizyphi Jujubae (*Da Zao*) to nourish the stomach. This results in *Si Qi Tang* (Four [Ingredients for the] Seven [Emotions] Decoction).

For chest oppression and fullness, add Tuber Curcumae (*Yu Jin*) and Fructus Citri Seu Ponciri (*Zhi Ke*).

For chest pain, add Fructus Trichosanthis Kirlowii (*Gua Lou*) and Bulbus Allii (*Xie Bai*).

For chest oppression and coughing, add Radix Bupleuri (*Chai Hu*), Radix Platycodi Grandiflori (*Jie Geng*), Cortex Radicis Mori (*Sang Bai Pi*), and Semen Pruni Armeniacae (*Xing Ren*).

For ulcers, add Radix Panacis Ginseng (*Ren Shen*) and mix-fried Radix Glycyrrhizae (*Zhi Gan Cao*).

Also for ulcers, to the above add Cortex Cinnamomi (*Rou Gui*) and Radix Scutellariae Baicalensis (*Huang Qin*).

For abdominal distention, add Fructus Amomi (*Sha Ren*) and Radix Saussureae Seu Vladimiriae (*Mu Xiang*).

For hypochondrial and lateral costal pain, add Fructus Meliae Toosendan (*Chuan Lian Zi*) and Rhizoma Corydalis Yanhusuo (*Yan Hu*).

For pain and swelling of the throat, add Radix Scrophulariae Ningpoensis (*Yuan Shen*) and Radix Platycodi Grandiflori (*Jie Geng*).

10.2 *Jiang Qi Ji* (Downbearing qi formulas)

Representative formula: *Ju Pi Zhu Ru Tang* (Orange Peel & Caulis Bambusae Decoction)

Composition:

Pericarpium Citri Reticulatae (*Ju Pi*), 12g
Caulis In Taeniis Bambusae (*Zhu Ru*), 12g
Fructus Zizyphi Jujubae (*Da Zao*), 5 pieces
raw Rhizoma Zingiberis (*Sheng Jiang*), 9g

163

Radix Glycyrrhizae (*Gan Cao*), 6g
Radix Panacis Ginseng (*Ren Shen*), 3g

Functions: Downbears counterflow and stops hiccup, boosts the qi and clears heat

Indications: Qi vacuity with heat, qi counterflow and no downbearing. Hiccup, nausea and vomiting, morning sickness, post-surgical persistent hiccup, chronic gastric diseases, and incomplete pyloric obstruction

Main signs & symptoms: Hiccup, nausea, dry heaves, a tender, red tongue, and a thready, rapid or vacuous, rapid pulse

Contraindications:

1. Do not use for hiccup or vomiting due to replete heat.
2. Do not use for hiccup or vomiting due to vacuity cold.

Formula explanation:

Within this formula, Orange Peel and Caulis Bambusae are the sovereign medicinals. Orange Peel moves the qi and harmonizes the stomach, thus stopping hiccup. Caulis Bambusae clears heat and quiets the stomach, thus stopping hiccup. They are both used in relatively large amounts in this formula. Ginseng supplements the qi and supports the righteous. When combined with Orange Peel, these two both move and supplement the center. Fresh Ginger harmonizes the stomach and stops vomiting. Combined with Caulis Bambusae, these two clear but also warm the center. Ginseng and Ginger are the minister medicinals in this formula. Licorice and Red Dates assist Ginseng in boosting the qi and harmonizing the stomach. Being regulating medicinals, they are the assistants and messengers within this prescription. Taken as a whole, this formula supplements stomach vacuity, clears stomach heat, and downbears stomach counterflow.

Thus it supplements with causing stagnation and clears with causing cold. It is appropriate to use when there is both stomach vacuity and heat causing hiccup, vomiting, and dry heaves.

Additions & subtractions:

For concomitant phlegm, add Sclerotium Poriae Cocos (*Fu Ling*) and Rhizoma Pinelliae Ternatae (*Ban Xia*).

For concomitant stomach yin vacuity, add Tuber Ophiopogonis Japonicae (*Mai Dong*) and Herba Dendrobii (*Shi Hu*).

Also for stomach yin vacuity, add Tuber Ophiopogonis Japonicae (*Mai Dong*), Radix Glehniae Littoralis (*Sha Shen*), Rhizoma Phragmitis Communis (*Lu Gen*), and Folium Eriobotryae Japonicae (*Pi Pa Ye*).

For less obvious or no concomitant qi vacuity, subtract Ginseng.

For vomiting or hiccup due to stomach yin vacuity and disharmony, add Sclerotium Poriae Cocos (*Fu Ling*), Rhizoma Pinelliae Ternatae (*Ban Xia*), Tuber Ophiopogonis Japonicae (*Mai Dong*), and Folium Eriobotryae Japonicae (*Pi Pa Ye*). This results in *Ji Sheng Ju Pi Zhu Ru Tang* (Aiding Life Orange Peel & Caulis Bambusae Decoction).

For vomiting due to stomach heat, subtract Ginseng, Licorice, and Red Dates and add Calyx Kaki Diospyros (*Shi Di*). This results in *Xin Zhi Ju Pi Zhu Ru Tang* (Newly Processed Orange Peel and Caulis Bambusae Decoction).

Comment: For the treatment of morning sickness, this decoction can be given by drops on the tongue throughout the day.

小青龍湯治水氣
喘咳嘔噦渴利慰
薑桂麻黃芍藥甘
細辛半夏兼五味

Mnemonic verse for learning *Xiao Qing Long Tang*

11

Li Xue Ji
Rectifying the Blood Formulas

Formulas which rectify the blood are divided into two subcategories: 1) formulas which quicken the blood and dispel stasis, and 2) formulas which stop bleeding. Blood stasis may be due to prolonged qi depression, cold, heat, or trauma. It may also be categorized as replete or vacuous, mild or severe, acute or chronic. In addition, treatment typically takes into account the location of the stasis. Blood-quickening, stasis-dispelling formulas are commonly used in internal medicine, gynecology, traumatology, and in external medicine.

Stop-bleeding formulas are used in all sorts of hemorrhagic disorders. Bleeding may be due to only four disease mechanisms in TCM. First, heat may cause the blood to flow recklessly outside its pathways. Evil heat causing bleeding may be further divided between replete heat, vacuity heat, depressive heat, and damp or phlegm heat. Secondly, stasis may force the blood outside its pathways. Third, qi may be too vacuous to restrain the blood within its channels. Fourth, traumatic injury may rupture the channels and vessels, so the blood cannot be canalized and flow freely. Under the stop-bleeding category of formulas, most formulas stop bleeding by either clearing heat or supplementing vacuity.

Cautions & Contraindications:

1. Hemostatic medicinals may cause stasis if used in too large doses, for too long a time, or unwarrantedly.

2. Blood-quickening, stasis-dispelling medicinals are attacking in nature. Therefore, if they are used in too large a dose or for too long a time, they can consume blood and yin.
3. In case of blood desertion, first supplement the qi greatly before using hemostatic medicinals.
4. If blood stasis complicates or is causing bleeding, one must use blood-quickening medicinals *in order* to help stop bleeding.

11.1 *Huo Xue Zhu Yu Ji* (Blood-quickening, stasis-dispelling formulas)

Representative formulas:

A. *Xue Fu Zhu Yu Tang* (Dispelling Stasis from the Blood Mansion Decoction)

Composition:

Semen Pruni Persicae (*Tao Ren*), 12g
Flos Carthami Tinctorii (*Tao Ren*), 9g
Radix Angelicae Sinensis (*Dang Gui*), 9g
raw Radix Rehmanniae (*Sheng Di*), 9g
Rhizoma Ligustici Wallichii (*Chuan Xiong*), 5g
Radix Rubrus Paeoniae Lactiflorae (*Chi Shao*), 6g
Radix Achyranthis Bidentatae (*Niu Xi*), 9g
Radix Platycodi Grandiflori (*Jie Geng*), 5g
Radix Bupleuri (*Chai Hu*), 3g
Fructus Citri Seu Ponciri (*Zhi Ke*), 6g
Radix Glycyrrhizae (*Gan Cao*), 3g

Functions: Quickens the blood and dispels stasis, moves the qi and stops pain

Indications: Blood stasis in the chest, blood not moving smoothly. Coronary heart disease, angina pectoris, rheumatic heart disease, intercostal neuralgia, costochondritis, functional neurosis, post-concussion syndrome, migraine, trigeminal neuralgia, external injury to the chest, irregular menstruation, dysmenorrhea, menopausal syndrome, cerebral hemorrhage, hypertension, cor pulmonale, and urticaria

Main signs & symptoms: Chest pain, headache which does not heal for many days, pain like a needle prick, possible hiccup for many days which will not stop, a choking sensation when drinking water, dry heaves, internal heat and oppression, possible heart palpitations, possible inability to sleep at night or one's sleep is not quiet, tension, agitation, easy anger, tidal fever, a dark red tongue, possible static patches or spots on the tongue, dark lips or dark around the eyes, and a choppy or wiry, tight pulse

Contraindications:

1. Do not use during pregnancy.
2. Do not use for uterine bleeding or other hemorrhagic disorders.

Formula explanation:

Within this formula, *Tao Hong Si Wu Tang* (Persica & Carthamus Four Materials Decoction) quickens the blood, transforms stasis, and also nourishes the blood, while *Si Ni San* (Four Counterflows Powder) moves the qi, harmonizes the blood, and soothes the liver. Platycodon opens the lung qi and guides the other medicinals upward. Combined with Citrus, these two upbear and downbear the qi of the upper burner and loosen the chest. Achyranthis opens and disinhibits the blood vessels and leads the qi to move downward. Taken as a whole, this formula quickens the blood and moves the qi, transforms phlegm and disperses heat while it also resolves depression of the liver.

169

Additions & subtractions:

For headache, add Fructus Viticis (*Man Jing Zi*) and Fructus Tribuli Terrestris (*Bai Ji Li*).

For pain in the hypochondrium and lateral costal regions, add Tuber Curcumae (*Yu Jin*) and Bulbus Allii (*Xie Bai*).

For immobile subcostal and abdominal masses, add Tuber Curcumae (*Yu Jin*) and Radix Salviae Miltiorrhizae (*Dan Shen*).

For gynecological conditions, such as amenorrhea or dysmenorrhea, subtract Platycodon and add Rhizoma Cyperi Rotundi (*Xiang Fu*), Herba Leonuri Heterophylli (*Yi Mu Cao*), and Herba Lycopi Lucidi (*Ze Lan*).

Also for gynecological conditions, subtract Platycodon and add Rhizoma Cyperi Rotundi (*Xiang Fu*), Herba Leonuri Heterophylli (*Yi Mu Cao*), and Radix Linderae Strychnifoliae (*Wu Yao*).

For angina pectoris, increase the dosages of Carthamus and Ligusticum and add Radix Salviae Miltiorrhizae (*Dan Shen*).

B. *Shi Xiao San* (Loss of Smile Powder)

Composition:

Feces Trogopterori Seu Pteromi (*Wi Ling Zhi*), 15g
Pollen Typhae (*Pu Huang*), 15g, stir-fried until aromatic

Functions: Quickens the blood and dispels stasis, scatters nodulation and stops pain

Indications: Blood stasis, stoppage, and stagnation. Retention of lochia, dysmenorrhea, angina pectoris, amenorrhea, irregular menstruation, postpartum abdominal pain, and endometriosis

Main signs & symptoms: Lancinating pain in the heart or abdomen, possible postpartum non-movement of the lochia, possible menstrual irregularity, lower abdominal tension and pain, a dark red tongue with possible static patches or spots, a choppy, wiry, or knotted (*i.e.*, bound) pulse

Contraindications:

1. Do not use during pregnancy.
2. Use with care in cases with stomach vacuity.

Formula explanation:

In this formula, Feces Trogopterori and Pollen Typhae work together to open and disinhibit the blood vessels, dispel stasis and stop pain.

Additions & subtractions:

For liver depression, qi stagnation, add Fructus Meliae Toosendan (*Chuan Lian Zi*) and Rhizoma Cyperi Rotundi (*Xiang Fu*).

For cold pain, add Radix Angelicae Sinensis (*Dang Gui*) and Folium Artemisiae Argyii (*Ai Ye*).

Also for concomitant cold, add blast-fried Rhizoma Zingiberis (*Pao Jiang*), Folium Artemisiae Argyii (*Ai Ye*), Fructus Foeniculi Vulgaris (*Xiao Hui Xiang*), and Radix Linderae Strychnifoliae (*Wu Yao*).

For irregular menstruation due to a combination of blood stasis and blood vacuity, add *Si Wu Tang* (Four Materials Decoction), *i.e.*, Radix Angelicae Sinensis (*Dang Gui*), Radix Albus Paeoniae Lactiflorae (*Bai*

171

Shao), prepared Radix Rehmanniae (*Shu Di*), and Rhizoma Ligustici Wallichii (*Chuan Xiang*).

For angina pectoris due to blood stasis, add Rhizoma Ligustici Wallichii (*Chuan Xiong*), Radix Rubrus Paeoniae Lactiflorae (*Chi Shao*), Flos Carthami Tinctorii (*Hong Hua*), and Radix Salviae Miltiorrhizae (*Dan Shen*).

For postpartum chest and/or abdominal pain, add Fructus Crataegi (*Shan Zha*).

Comment: This formula is most often added to other formulas for severe dysmenorrhea due to blood stasis.

C. *Sheng Hua Tang* (Engendering & Transforming Decoction)

Composition:

Radix Angelicae Sinensis (*Quan Dang Gui*), 25g
Rhizoma Ligustici Wallichii (*Chuan Xiong*), 9g
Semen Pruni Persicae (*Tao Ren*), 6g, remove the skin and tip
dry Rhizoma Zingiberis (*Gan Jiang*), 2g, blast-fried till blackened
Radix Glycyrrhizae (*Gan Cao*), 2g, mix-fried

Method of preparation: Decoct with rice wine, rice wine and water, or simply water.

Functions: Quickens the blood and transforms stasis, warms the channels and stops pain

Indications: Postpartum blood vacuity contracting cold. Retention of lochia, retention of placental fragments, and numerous other postpartum complaints associated with malign blood retained in the lower abdomen and then possibly thrusting here and there, chronic endometritis, puerperal infection, and trichomonas vaginitis

Main signs & symptoms: Retention of lochia, lower abdominal chilly pain which dislikes pressure, dark, purplish lochia containing clots, a pale, purplish tongue with possible static patches or spots, and a fine, deep, choppy pulse

Contraindications:

1. Do not use during pregnancy.
2. Do not use for hemorrhagic disorders.
3. Do not use in cases of blood stasis due to heat in the blood.

Formula explanation:

Within this formula, a large dose of *Dang Gui* is the sovereign medicinal. It supplements and activates the blood, transforms stasis and generates new (*i.e.*, new blood). Ligusticum quickens the blood and moves the qi. Persica quickens the blood and dispels stasis. These are the two minister medicinals. Blast-fried Ginger enters the blood and scatters cold, warms the channels and stops pain. Rice Wine warms and opens the blood vessels, thus assisting the power of the other medicinals. Mix-fried Licorice regulates and harmonizes all these other medicinals and is the messenger medicinal in this prescription. Together, this formula nourishes the blood and transforms stasis, warms the channels and stops pain. It helps the lochia move smoothly and also cures lower abdominal chilly pain.

Additions & subtractions:

For severe cold, add Fructus Foeniculi Vulgaris (*Xiao Hui Xiang*) and Cortex Cinnamomi (*Rou Gui*).

173

For even more severe cold, add Radix Praeparatus Aconiti Carmi-chaeli (*Fu Zi*) and Cortex Cinnamomi (*Rou Gui*).

For severe abdominal pain due to static blood, add *Shi Xiao San* (Loss of Smile Powder), see above, and Rhizoma Corydalis Yanhusuo (*Yan Hu*).

Also for severe abdominal pain due to stasis, add Pollen Typhae (*Pu Huang*), Rhizoma Corydalis Yanhusuo (*Yan Hu*), and Herba Leonuri Heterophylli (*Yi Mu Cao*).

If the lochia is almost finished or the pain associated with the lochia is mild, subtract Persica.

For concomitant qi vacuity, add Radix Panacis Ginseng (*Ren Shen*) and Radix Astragali Membranacei (*Huang Qi*).

If heat is transformed from prolonged stasis, subtract blast-fried Ginger and add Radix Rubrus Paeoniae Lactiflorae (*Chi Shao*) and Cortex Radicis Moutan (*Dan Pi*).

For puerperal fever due to blood stasis, subtract Licorice and add Radix Salviae Miltiorrhizae (*Dan Shen*), Cortex Radicis Moutan (*Dan Pi*), and Radix Rubrus Paeoniae Lactiflorae (*Chi Shao*) to quicken the blood and recede fever.

For failure of the uterus to resume its normal size, add Herba Leonuri Heterophylli (*Yi Mu Cao*).

For abnormal vaginal discharge with a bloody, mucoid discharge, pain in the lower abdomen, a purple tongue, and a choppy pulse, subtract Licorice and add Herba Lycopi Lucidi (*Ze Lan*) to quicken the blood and dispel stasis.

11.2 *Zhi Xue Ji* (Stop-bleeding formulas)

Representative formulas:

A. *Shi Hui San* (Ten Ashes Powder)

Composition:

Herba Cirsii (*Da Ji*)
Herba Cephalanoplos (*Xiao Ji*)
Folium Nelumbinis Nuciferae (*He Ye*)
Cacumen Biotae Orientalis (*Ce Bai Ye*)
Rhizoma Imperatae Cylindricae (*Mao Gen*)
Radix Rubiae Cordifoliae (*Qian Cao*)
Fructus Gardeniae Jasminoidis (*Shan Zhi*)
Radix Et Rhizoma Rhei (*Da Huang*)
Cortex Radicis Moutan (*Dan Pi*)
Fibra Stipulae Trachycarpi (*Zong Lu Pi*)

Method of preparation & administration: Carbonize equal parts of the above medicinals in a sealed container and then grind into a fine powder. Take 9-15g of this powder made into pills mixed with ink made from a Chinese inkstick ground in either lotus root juice or white radish juice. However, this powder can also be added to other formulas as a heat-clearing hemostatic ingredient. It can also be prepared as a decoction on its own.

Functions: Cools the blood and stops bleeding

Indications: Blood heat reckless movement, replete fire in the liver and stomach. Hematemesis, hemoptysis, epistaxis, pulmonary tuberculosis, bronchiectasis, acute hemorrhagic esophagitis or gastritis, peptic ulcer bleeding, hemorrhagic febrile diseases, and functional uterine bleeding

Main signs & symptoms: Acute onset vomiting, coughing or spitting up blood, or nosebleed, a red tongue, and a replete, rapid pulse

Contraindications:

1. Do not use for vacuity bleeding patterns.
2. Do not use for cold bleeding patterns.

Formula explanation:

Within this formula, Cirsium, Cephalanoplos, Lotus Leaf, Rubia, Cacumen Biotae, and Imperata all cool the blood and stop bleeding. Trachycarpus restrains and astringes and stops bleeding. Gardenia clears heat and drains fire, while Rhubarb leads away heat and moves it downward. Thus these two ingredients help the others by downbearing fire. Moutan combined with Rhubarb cools the blood and dispels stasis, thus this combination helps cool the blood and stop bleeding without retaining stasis. The ingredients in this formula are preferably used carbonized since this strengthens their ability to restrain, astringe, and stop bleeding. Lotus Root or Radish Root Juice mixed with ink also helps strengthen the heat-clearing, blood-cooling, and stop bleeding functions of the above medicinals.

Comment: When this formula is prepared as a decoction, its ability to clear heat and conduct it downward is even stronger.

B. *Huang Tu Tang* (Yellow Earth Decoction)

Composition:

Radix Glycyrrhizae (*Gan Cao*), 9g
dry Radix Rehmanniae (*Gan Di Huang*), 9g
Rhizoma Atractylodis Macrocephalae (*Bai Zhu*), 9g
Radix Praeparatus Aconiti Carmichaeli (*Fu Zi*), 9g, blast-fried

176

Gelatinum Corii Asini (*E Jiao*), 9g
Radix Scutellariae Baicalensis (*Huang Qin*), 9g
Terra Flava Usta (*Zao Xin Huang Tu*), 30g

Functions: Warms yang and fortifies the spleen, nourishes the blood and stops bleeding

Indications: Spleen yang insufficiency, middle burner vacuity cold. Chronic hemorrhagic gastritis, peptic ulcer bleeding, functional uterine bleeding

Main signs & symptoms: Hemafecia, hematemesis, epistaxis, or women's flooding and leaking, the color of the blood dull and pale, lack of warmth in the four extremities, a faded, yellow facial color, a pale tongue with a white coating, and a deep, fine, forceless pulse

Formula explanation:

Terra Flava Usta (also called *Fu Long Gan*) warms the center and stops bleeding. It is the sovereign medicinal in this formula. The combination of Atractylodis and Aconite warms spleen yang and supplements the central qi. These assist the sovereign medicinal in gaining control over the absorption of the blood and are the minister medicinals. However, the acrid warmth of Atractylodis and the Aconite's tendency to consume the blood and make it run reckless might otherwise result in excessive bleeding and cause yin and blood debility and consumption. Therefore, they are assisted by raw Rehmannia and Donkey Skin Glue to enrich yin and nourish the blood while at the same time stopping bleeding. When the bitter cold of Scutellaria is combined with the sweet, cold, and moistening of raw Rehmannia and Donkey Skin Glue, these control even further the warm, dry nature of Atractylodis and Aconite. On the other hand, Atractylodis and Aconite prevent the Rehmannia and Donkey Skin Glue from causing stagnation due to their being enriching and greasy.

177

Licorice regulates all these medicinals and harmonizes the center. It is the messenger medicinal.

Additions & subtractions:

In order to make this formula's ability to stop bleeding stronger, replace Scutellaria with carbonized Radix Scutellariae Baicalensis (*Huang Qin Tan*).

If bleeding is very excessive, add Pulvis Radicis Pseudoginseng (*San Qi Fen*, taken separately), Folium Artemisiae Argyii (*Ai Ye*), and blast-fried Rhizoma Zingiberis (*Pao Jiang*).

Also for excessive bleeding, add Pulvis Radicis Pseudoginseng (*San Qi Fen*), Rhizoma Bletillae Striatae (*Bai Ji*), and Folium Artemisiae Argyii (*Ai Ye*).

Yet another variation for excessive bleeding is to add Pulvis Radicis Pseudoginseng (*San Qi Fen*), Rhizoma Bletillae Striatae (*Bai Ji*), and Os Sepiae Seu Sepiellae (*Wu Zei Gu*).

If there is concomitant qi vacuity add Radix Panacis Ginseng (*Ren Shen*) and Radix Astragali Membranacei (*Huang Qi*).

For blood vacuity, add Arillus Euphoriae Longanae (*Long Yan Rou*) and Radix Angelicae Sinensis (*Dang Gui*).

For loose stools, replace Scutellaria with stir-fried Radix Scutellariae Baicalensis (*Chao Huang Qin*) and add blast-fried Rhizoma Zingiberis (*Pao Jiang*).

12

Zhi Feng Ji
Wind-treating Formulas

The formulas in this category are mostly composed of either acrid, scattering medicinals which expel wind or ingredients which extinguish wind and stop tetany. The first group course and scatter external wind, while the second group level and extinguish internal wind. Thus the treatment of wind comprises these two subdivisions of formulas. External wind is due to wind evils entering into the human body from the outside. These may enter the flesh, channels, sinews, joints, or bones and give rise to rashes, dizziness, numbness, difficulty moving, and joint pain. It is also possible for external wind to cause the movement of internal wind, giving rise to muscular tetany, clenched jaws, opisthotonos, facial paralysis, and other disorders characterized by spasming of the muscles.

Internal wind is due to the stirring of liver wind internally. This in turn is most often due to liver/kidney dual vacuity and ascendancy of liver yang. Internal wind may also be generated by extreme internal heat. The signs and symptoms of stirring of internal wind include headache, dizziness, blurred vision, tinnitus, and muscle twitching. When extreme, stirring of internal wind may give rise to wind stroke with sudden loss of consciousness, paralysis, tetany, and aphasia. It should be remembered that internal wind is nothing other than counterflowing yang qi moving recklessly and moving upward and outward. Thus formulas for internal wind often include blood-nourishing and yin-enriching medicinals.

Other formulas which treat wind may be found under other categories, such as exterior-relieving formulas and dispelling wind, overcoming dampness formulas.

12.1 *Shu San Wai Feng Ji* (Coursing & scattering external wind formulas)

Representative formula: *Chuan Xiong Chao Tiao San* (Ligusticum & Tea Regulating Powder)

Composition:

Rhizoma Ligustici Wallichii (*Chuan Xiong*), 9g
Herba Seu Flos Schizonepetae Tenuifoliae (*Jing Jie*), 9g
Radix Angelicae (*Bai Zhi*), 6g
Radix Et Rhizoma Notopterygii (*Qiang Huo*), 6g
Radix Glycyrrhizae (*Gan Cao*), 6g
Herba Cum Radice Asari (*Xi Xin*), 3g
Radix Ledebouriellae Sesloidis (*Fang Feng*), 4.5g
Herba Menthae (*Bo He*), 6g, do not allow to see fire, *i.e.*, do not decoct, only steep

Method of preparation: Decoct the first seven ingredients for not more than 10 minutes and then add the Mint and Folium Camelliae Theae (*Qing Cha*, Green Tea) and allow to steep.

Functions: Courses wind and stops pain

Indications: External invasion of wind evils headache. Common cold and flus with headache, migraines, tension headache, neurogenic headache, acute and chronic rhinitis and sinusitis, vertigo

Main signs & symptoms: Headache in any part of the head accompanied by fever, aversion to wind and cold, fever, possible dizziness, nasal congestion, a thin, white tongue coating, and a floating, tight pulse

Contraindications:

1. Do not use to treat liver yang ascendant or liver/kidney dual vacuity, *i.e.*, yin vacuity, headache.
2. Do not use to treat qi and blood vacuity headache.

Formula explanation:

Within this formula, Ligusticum, Angelica, and Notopterygium course wind and stop pain. Ligusticum has an affinity for treating *shao yin* and *jue yin* channel headaches. Notopterygium has an affinity for treating *tai yang* channel headaches, and Angelica has an affinity for treating *yang ming* channel headaches. These are the sovereign medicinals in this prescription. Asarum scatters cold and stops pain. It is able to treat *shao yin* channel headache. Mint is able to clear and disinhibit the head and eyes. It tracks down wind and scatters heat. Schizonepeta and Ledebouriella are acrid, scattering, and move upward. They course and scatter wind evils from the upper parts. Each of these medicinals assist the sovereign medicinal and strengthen the coursing of wind and stopping of pain. They are also able to relieve the exterior and are the minister medicinals. Licorice regulates and harmonizes all these other medicinals. It is used occasionally with Green Tea in order to regulate its precipitation. Green Tea's nature and flavor are bitter and cold. Thus, it is able to clear the head and eyes above. Together, these two are able to restrain the other warm, drying, upbearing, and scattering medicinals. Therefore, these two are the assistant and messenger medicinals.

Additions & subtractions:

For wind cold headache or marked aversion to cold, subtract Mint and add raw Rhizoma Zingiberis (*Sheng Jiang*) and Folium Perillae Frutescentis (*Su Ye*).

For wind heat headache with a yellow coated tongue and a rapid pulse, subtract Notopterygium and Asarum and add Flos Chrysanthemi Morifolii (*Ju Hua*), Fructus Viticis (*Man Jing Zi*), and Ramulus Uncariae Cum Uncis (*Gou Teng*).

For chronic rhinitis and nasal sinusitis, add Flos Magnoliae (*Xin Yi Hua*) and Fructus Xanthii (*Cang Er Zi*).

For headache due to wind heat with dizziness and vertigo, add Flos Chrysanthemi Morifolii (*Ju Hua*), Bombyx Batryticatus (*Jiang Can*), and mix-fried Radix Glycyrrhizae (*Zhi Gan Cao*). This results in *Ju Hua Cha Tiao San* (Chrysanthemum & Tea Regulating Powder).

For chronic headache complicated by blood stasis, add Flos Carthami Tinctorii (*Hong Hua*), Semen Pruni Persicae (*Tao Ren*), Bombyx Batryticatus (*Jiang Can*), and Buthus Martensis (*Quan Xie*).

For headache predominately along the course of the *tai yang*, add Radix Et Rhizoma Ligustici Chinensis (*Gao Ben*).

For headache predominately along the course of the *shao yang*, add Radix Bupleuri (*Chai Hu*).

For headache predominately along the course of the *yang ming*, add Radix Puerariae Lobatae (*Ge Gen*).

For headaches predominately at the vertex, *i.e.*, along the course of the *jue yin*, add Fructus Evodiae Rutecarpae (*Wu Zhu Yu*) and Lumbricus (*Di Long*).

12.2 *Ping Xi Nei Feng Ji* (Levelling & extinguishing internal wind formulas)

Representative formulas:

A. *Zhen Gan Xi Feng Tang* (Settle the Liver & Extinguish Wind Decoction)

Composition:

Radix Achyranthis Bidentatae (*Huai Niu Xi*), 30g
Haemititum (*Dai Zhe Shi*), 30g
raw Os Draconis (*Sheng Long Gu*), 15g
raw Concha Ostreae (*Sheng Mu Li*), 15g
raw Plastrum Testudinis (*Sheng Gui Ban*), 15g
raw Radix Albus Paeoniae Lactiflorae (*Sheng Hang Yao*), 15g
Radix Scrophulariae Ningpoensis (*Yuan Shen*), 15g
Tuber Asparagi Cochinensis (*Tian Dong*), 15g
Fructus Meliae Toosendan (*Chuan Lian Zi*), 6g
raw Fructus Germinatus Hordei Vulgaris (*Sheng Mai Ya*), 6g
Herba Artemisiae Capillaris (*Yin Chen*), 6g
Radix Glycyrrhizae (*Gan Cao*), 4.5g

Functions: Settles the liver and extinguishes wind, enriches yin and subdues yang

Indications: Liver/kidney yin deficiency, liver yang ascendancy, qi and blood counterflow and chaos. Wind stroke, convulsions, epilepsy, cerebrovascular accident, aphasia, apraxia, renal hypertension, essential hypertension, hypertensive encephalopathy, cerebral arteriosclerosis, arteriosclerotic heart disease, hyperthyroidism, premenstrual tension, postpartum fever with spasms and convulsions, and glaucoma

Main signs & symptoms: Headache, dizziness, vertigo, distention of the eyes, tinnitus, hot pain in the brain region, vexatious heat within the heart, a facial color as if drunk (*i.e.*, flushed), frequent belching, inability to control the limbs of the body, deviation of the eyes and mouth, if serious, dizziness and vertigo leading to collapse, loss of consciousness of human affairs, essence spirit short and scant, and a long, wiry, forceful pulse

Contraindications:

1. Use with care and/or modification in patients with spleen vacuity.

Formula explanation:

Within this formula, Achyranthis restores the liver/kidney channels and conducts the blood to move downward. It also supplements and boosts the liver and kidneys. It is the sovereign medicinal in this prescription. Hematite, Dragon Bone, and Oyster Shell downbear counterflow and subdue yang. They settle and extinguish liver wind and are the minister medicinals. Plastrum Testudinis, Scrophularia, Asparagus, and White Peony enrich and nourish yin fluids. Thus they control yang hyperactivity. Artemisia Capillaris, Melia, and Malted Barley, when combined with the sovereign medicinal, clear and drain surplus of liver yang and out-thrust liver qi depression and stagnation. Thus these ingredients disinhibit liver yang by levelling, resolving, settling, and subduing. Licorice regulates and harmonizes all these other medicinals. Combined with Malted Barley, these two are also able to harmonize the stomach and regulate the center. These are the assistant and messenger medicinals.

Additions & subtractions:

For headache, blurred vision, vertigo, and dizziness, add Spica Prunellae Vulgaris (*Xia Gu Cao*) and Flos Chrysanthemi Morifolii (*Ju Hua*).

For severe distention and pain in the eyes, add Spica Prunellae Vulgaris (*Xia Gu Cao*) and Concha Haliotidis (*Shi Jue Ming*).

Also for severe distention and pain in the eyes, add Ramulus Uncariae Cum Uncis (*Gou Teng*) and Flos Chrysanthemi Morifolii (*Ju Hua*).

And again, for severe pain and distention in the eyes, add Pulvus Cornu Antelopis (*Ling Yang Fen*).

For excessive phlegm, subtract Licorice and Scrophularia and add bile-processed Rhizoma Arisaematis (*Dan Nan Xing*) and Bulbus Fritillariae Cirrhosae (*Chuan Bei Mu*).

If there is concomitant kidney vacuity, add prepared Radix Rehmanniae (*Shu Di*) and Fructus Corni Officinalis (*Shan Zhu Yu*).

If there is a weak *chi* pulse, subtract Melia and add Fructus Corni Officinalis (*Shan Zhu Yu*) to enrich and supplement the liver and kidneys.

If there is concomitant vexatious heat in the heart, add raw Gypsum (*Sheng Shi Gao*) and Fructus Gardeniae Jasminoidis (*Shan Zhi Zi*).

For loose stools, subtract Plastrum Testudinis and Hematite and add Hallyositum Rubrum (*Chi Shi Zhi*).

For postpartum fever with spasms and convulsions, a red tongue, and a rapid, wiry pulse, add Fructus Chaenomelis Lagenariae (*Mu Gua*) and Ramulus Uncariae Cum Uncis (*Gou Teng*).

For hypertension, add Spica Prunellae Vulgaris (*Xia Gu Cao*), Ramulus Uncariae Cum Uncis (*Gou Teng*), and Flos Chrysanthemi Morifolii (*Ju Hua*).

For cerebral arteriosclerosis, add Concha Haliotidis (*Shi Jue Ming*), Rhizoma Atractylodis (*Cang Zhu*), Pericarpium Citri Reticulatae (*Chen Pi*), Semen Pruni Persicae (*Tao Ren*), and Herba Agastachis Seu Pogostemi (*Huo Xiang*).

For arteriosclerotic heart disease, add Radix Rubrus Paeoniae Lactiflorae (*Chi Shao*) and Radix Salviae Miltiorrhizae (*Dan Shen*).

B. *Tian Ma Gou Teng Yin* (Gastrodia & Uncaria Drink)

Composition:

Rhizoma Gastrodiae Elatae (*Tian Ma*), 9g
Ramulus Uncariae Cum Uncis (*Gou Teng*), 12g, added after
Concha Haliotidis (*Shi Jue Ming*), 18g, decocted before
Fructus Gardeniae Jasminoidis (*Shan Zhi*), 9g
Radix Scutellariae Baicalensis (*Huang Qin*), 9g
Radix Cyathulae (*Chuan Niu Xi*), 12g
Cortex Eucommiae Ulmoidis (*Du Zhong*), 9g
Herba Leonuri Heterophylli (*Yi Mu Cao*), 9g
Ramulus Loranthi Seu Visci (*Sang Ji Sheng*), 9g
Caulis Polygoni Multiflori (*Ye Jiao Teng*), 9g
Cinnabar(-processed) Sclerotium Pararadicis Poriae Cocos (*Zhu Fu Shen*), 9g

Functions: Levels the liver and extinguishes wind, clears heat and quickens the blood, and supplements and boosts the liver and kidneys

Indications: Ascendant liver yang, liver wind harassing above. Cerebrovascular disease, transitory ischemic attacks, hemiplegia, essential hypertension, renal hypertension, hypertensive encephalopathy, aphasia, apraxia, epilepsy, puerperal eclampsia, trigeminal neuralgia, and neurosis

Main signs & symptoms: Headache, dizziness, vertigo, insomnia, paralysis or convulsions, deviation of the mouth and eyes, a quivering, red tongue, and a wiry, rapid pulse

Formula explanation:

In this formula, Gastrodia, Uncaria, and Abalone Shell level the liver and extinguish wind. They are the sovereign medicinals. Gardenia and Scutellaria clear heat and drain fire. Therefore, they assist in keeping liver channel heat from ascending upward. These are the minister medicinals. Leonurus quickens the blood and disinhibits water. Cyathula conducts the blood and moves it downward. Eucommmia and Loranthus combined together are able to supplement and boost the liver and kidneys. Caulis Polygoni Multiflori and Cinnabar-processed Spirit of Poria quiet the spirit and tranquilize the orientation (*i.e.*, emotions). These are the assistant and messenger medicinals.

Additions & subtractions:

If the disease is serious, add Cornu Antelopis (*Ling Yang Jiao*).

参苓白术扁豆陈

山药甘莲砂薏仁

桔梗上浮姜保婶

枣汤调服善醒神

Mnemonic verse for learning *Shen Lin Bai Zhu San*

13

Zhi Zao Ji
Treating Dryness Formulas

This category of formulas is composed of formulas which treat externally contracted dryness and those which treat internal dryness due to yin vacuity. The former subcategory of formulas uses medicinals which gently diffuse dry evils, while the latter are composed of medicinals which enrich yin and moisten dryness. External dryness is primarily due to external invasion by dry evils. These evils may combine with wind or cold and may easily transform into heat or fire. Internal dryness is due to essence deficiency and fluid consumption of the viscera and bowels. In turn, this may be due to excessive loss of body fluids through vomiting, sweating, or diarrhea, excessive urination, sexual taxation, or overindulgence in spicy foods. The lungs, spleen, kidneys, and large intestine are the viscera and bowels most commonly affected by fluid dryness.

Cautions & Contraindications:

1. Do not use moistening, enriching formulas with patients who have a damp body constitution.
2. Use with care in cases of diarrhea due to spleen vacuity.
3. Use with care in cases of qi stagnation since greasy, enriching, and supplementing ingredients can further obstruct the free flow of qi.

13.1 *Ruan Xuan Ru Zao Ji* (Mildly diffusing & moistening dryness formulas)

Representative formula: *Xing Su San* (Armeniaca & Perilla Powder)

Composition:

Folium Perillae Frutescentis (*Su Ye*), 6g
Rhizoma Pinelliae Ternatae (*Ban Xia*), 6g
Sclerotium Poriae Cocos (*Fu Ling*), 6g
Radix Peucedani (*Qian Hu*), 6g
Radix Platycodi Grandiflori (*Ku Jie Geng*), 6g
Fructus Citri Seu Ponciri (*Zhi Ke*), 6g
Radix Glycyrrhizae (*Gan Cao*), 6g
raw Rhizoma Zingiberis (*Sheng Jiang*), 6g
Pericarpium Citri Reticulatae (*Ju Pi*), 6g
Semen Pruni Armeniacae (*Xing Ren*), 6g
Fructus Zizyphi Jujubae (*Da Zao*), 2 pieces

Functions: Gently diffuses and cools dryness, diffuses the lungs and transforms phlegm

Indications: External invasion, cool dryness. Common cold, chronic tracheitis, acute and chronic bronchitis, bronchiectasis, and pulmonary emphysema

Main signs & symptoms: Slight headache, aversion to cold, no sweating, cough with sticky phlegm, stuffed nose, dry throat, a white tongue coating, and a wiry pulse

Formula explanation:

Within this formula, Folium Perillae and Peucedanum relieve the exterior and scatter evils as well as cause slight sweating. Armeniaca and Platycodon diffuse the lungs and out-thrust evils, disinhibit the qi and stop coughing. Pinellia and Poria dispel dampness and transform phlegm. Citrus and Orange Peel rectify the qi and loosen the chest. Fresh Ginger, Red Dates, and Licorice regulate the constructive and defensive and harmonize all the other medicinals. Taken as a whole, this formula emits the exterior, diffuses the lungs, and cools and resolves dryness. It also disinhibits the qi, transforms phlegm, and stops cough.

Additions & subtractions:

For severe aversion to cold, add Herba Allii Fistulosi (*Cong Bai*) and Semen Praeparatum Sojae (*Dan Dou Chi*).

For severe headache, add Rhizoma Ligustici Wallichii (*Chuan Xiong*) and Radix Ledebouriellae Sesloidis (*Fang Feng*).

For frontal headache above the eyes, add Radix Angelicae (*Bai Zhi*).

If there is no perspiration and a very wiry or tight pulse, add Radix Et Rhizoma Notopterygii (*Qiang Huo*).

For cough with copious phlegm, add Radix Asteris Tartarici (*Zi Wan*) and Bulbus Fritillariae (*Bei Mu*).

For cough with scant phlegm, subtract Pinellia and Poria.

For cough with copious phlegm, increase the dosages of Pinellia and Orange Peel.

If there is concomitant diarrhea and abdominal fullness, add Rhizoma Atractylodis (*Cang Zhu*) and Cortex Magnoliae Officinalis (*Hou Po*).

For simultaneous internal heat, add Radix Scutellariae Baicalensis (*Huang Qin*).

For simultaneous qi vacuity, add Radix Codonopsis Pilosulae (*Dang Shen*).

13.2 *Zi Yin Ru Zao Ji* (Enriching yin, moistening dryness formulas)

Representative formula: Bai He Gu Jin Tang (Bulbus Lilii Secure the Lungs Decoction)

Composition:

raw Radix Rehmanniae (*Sheng Di*), 6g
prepared Radix Rehmanniae (*Shu Di*), 9g
Tuber Ophiopogonis Japonicae (*Mai Dong*), 5g
Bulbus Lilii (*Bai He*), 3g
Radix Albus Paeoniae Lactiflorae (*Bai Shao*), 3g, stir-fried
Radix Angelicae Sinensis (*Dang Gui*), 3g
Bulbus Fritillariae (*Bei Mu*), 3g
raw Radix Glycyrrhizae (*Sheng Gan Cao*), 3g
Radix Scrophulariae Ningpoensis (*Xuan Shen*), 3g
Radix Platycodi Grandiflori (*Jie Geng*), 3g

Functions: Nourishes yin and moistens the lungs, transforms phlegm and stops cough

Indications: Lung/kidney yin vacuity. Chronic bronchitis, bronchiectasis, hemoptysis, chronic pharyngitis, laryngitis, polyps on the vocal cords, carcinoma of the larynx, spontaneous pneumothorax, cor pulmonale, silicosis, and pulmonary tuberculosis

Main signs & symptoms: Cough with bloody phlegm, dry painful throat, heat in the hands, feet, and heart, steaming bones, night sweats, a red tongue with scant coating, and a thready, rapid pulse

Contraindications:

1. Do not use unmodified in cases complicated by spleen vacuity.
2. Do not use unmodified in cases complicated by food stagnation.

Formula explanation:

In this formula, the two Rehmannias are the sovereigns. They enrich yin and supplement the kidneys. In particular, raw Rehmannia is also able to cool the blood and stop bleeding. Ophiopogon, Lily, and Fritillaria are the ministers. They moisten the lungs and nourish yin but are also able to transform phlegm and stop coughing. These are assisted by Scrophularia which enriches yin, cools the blood, and clears vacuity heat. Dang Gui nourishes the blood and moistens dryness. White Peony nourishes the blood and boosts yin. Platycodon diffuses and disinhibits the lung qi, stops coughing and transforms phlegm. Licorice is the messenger. It regulates and harmonizes all the other medicinals. Combined with Platycodon, these two disinhibit the throat.

Additions & subtractions:

For copious phlegm, add Fructus Trichosanthis (*Gua Lou*) and Cortex Radicis Mori (*Sang Pi*).

For constipation, add Semen Trichosanthis Kirlowii (*Gua Lou Ren*).

For hemoptysis, add Rhizoma Imperatae Cylindricae (*Bai Mao Gen*).

If coughing blood is excessive, subtract Platycodon and add Imperata and Herba Agrimoniae Pilosae (*Xian He Cao*).

For fever with dark yellow or green phlegm, add Rhizoma Anemarrhenae (*Zhi Mu*) and Herba Houttuyniae Cordatae (*Yu Xing Cao*).

For pulmonary tuberculosis with hemoptysis, add Tuber Bletillae Striatae (*Bai Ji*), Herba Agrimoniae Pilosae (*Xian He Cao*), and Herba Cum Radice Callicarpae Pedunculatae (*Zi Zhu Cao*).

For pulmonary tuberculosis with night sweats, malar flushing, vexatious heat, irritability, insomnia, nocturnal emissions, and shortness of breath, add Carapax Amydae (*Bie Jia*).

For lung cancer with yin vacuity, add Herba Houttuyniae Cordatae (*Yu Xing Cao*), Radix Rubrus Paeoniae Lactiflorae (*Chi Shao*), Herba Oldenlandiae (*Bai Hua She She Cao*), and Herba Scutellariae Barbatae (*Ban Zhi Lian*).

Comment: This formula should be used in combination with modern Western medicine when used to treat pulmonary tuberculosis.

14

Chu Shi Ji
Dispelling Dampness Formulas

The formulas in this category are primarily composed of dampness-dispelling medicinals which transform dampness and disinhibit water, free strangury and discharge turbidity. They treat water dampness disease. Because dampness is a yin evil whose nature is heavy and stagnant, in humans, damp diseases tend to progress slowly and also to linger. Damp evils may either enter the body from the outside or be internally generated. Externally contracted dampness may be due to lying in damp places, rainy weather, soaking in dampness, or getting wet from having sweat. Such external dampness mostly damages the muscles of the human body, the exterior, and the channels and network vessels. This results in aversion to cold, fever, heaviness and distention of the head, vexatious aching of the joints of the limbs, and possible facial and periocular edema.

Internal dampness is usually due to unrestrained eating of raw, chilled foods, excessive drinking of alcohol, and overthinking, worry, and anxiety. These result in damp turbidity becoming exuberant internally. In turn, this damages the spleen qi which loses its control over transportation and transformation. In this case, the manifestations typically include glomus and oppression of the chest and epigastrium, nausea, vomiting, diarrhea, jaundice, turbid strangury, edema of the lower legs and feet, etc. Because the muscles and exterior are connected with the viscera and bowels and the exterior and interior are mutually related, exterior dampness will eventually affect the viscera and bowels, while interior dampness may overflow outside into the muscles and skin. In that case, one may see manifestations of external and internal dampness occurring simultaneously.

External dampness is primarily treated by using the sweating method. Internal dampness is treated by any of several techniques. It may be aromatically transformed. One may use bitter warm medicinals to dry dampness, or one may use sweet, bland ingredients to disinhibit urination and percolate dampness. Each of these methods has its own uses and indications. In addition, if prolonged, dampness may be associated with cold. In that case, one must warm yang and transform dampness. Or, dampness, by impeding the free flow of yang qi, may become associated with heat. In that case, the heat must be cleared and the dampness eliminated.

There are five subcategories of damp-dispelling formulas: 1) Drying dampness, harmonizing the stomach formulas. This type of formula aromatically transforms dampness affecting the spleen/stomach and disturbing digestion. 2) Clearing heat, eliminating dampness formulas. These are used for various types of damp heat, such as damp heat jaundice, urinary and vaginal tract diseases, and foot qi. 3) Disinhibiting water, percolating dampness formulas. These are mostly used for treating urinary disturbances and edema. 4) Warm transforming water dampness formulas. These are used when dampness is associated with internal cold. 5) Dispelling wind, overcoming dampness formulas. These are used to treat wind dampness, *i.e.*, rheumatoid arthritic conditions.

Cautions & Contraindications

1. Use the formulas in this chapter with extreme caution in case of yin vacuity or consumption of fluids.
2. Because these formulas may be strongly attacking, they must be combined with righteous-supporting medicinals in those with bodily vacuity or during pregnancy.

14.1 *Zao Shi He Wei Ji* (Drying dampness, harmonizing the stomach formulas)

Representative formula: *Ping Wei San* (Levelling the Stomach Powder)

Composition:

Rhizoma Atractylodis (*Cang Zhu*), 9g
Cortex Magnoliae Officinalis (*Hou Po*), 9g
Pericarpium Citri Reticulatae (*Chen Pi*), 6g
Radix Glycyrrhizae (*Gan Cao*), 3g, stir-fried
raw Rhizoma Zingiberis (*Sheng Jiang*), 3g
Fructus Zizyphi Jujubae (*Da Zao*), 3 pieces

Functions: Dries dampness and transports the spleen, moves the qi and harmonizes the stomach

Indications: Damp stagnation of the spleen and stomach. Acute and chronic gastritis, gastrectasis, gastric ulcer, peptic ulcer, indigestion, especially pediatric indigestion, gastric neurosis, obesity, chronic pancreatitis, and parasitic diseases

Main signs & symptoms: Epigastric and abdominal distention and fullness, no thought of food or drink, a bland mouth and lack of taste, vomiting, nausea, acid eructation, a heavy, drooping feeling in the extremities, easy fatigue and a desire to lie down, a white, slimy or thick tongue coating, and a relaxed/retarded or possibly wiry pulse

Contraindications:

1. Use with caution during pregnancy.
2. Use with caution and/or modification in cases with yin and blood vacuity.

Formula explanation:

In this formula, a relatively large dose of Atractylodis is the sovereign. It is bitter, warm, and drying in nature. It is used to eliminate dampness and transport the spleen. Magnolia is the minister. It moves the qi and transforms dampness, disperses distention and eliminates fullness. Orange Peel is the assistant. It rectifies the qi and transforms stagnation. Licorice is the messenger. It is sweet and relaxing and harmonizes the stomach. It also regulates and harmonizes all the other medicinals. Fresh Ginger and Red Dates also regulate and harmonize the spleen and stomach. Therefore, the medicinals in this formula work together to transform damp turbidity, to regulate and smooth the qi dynamic, to augment and fortify the spleen and stomach, and to harmonize and downbear the stomach qi. Thus all the disease conditions associated with this formula are automatically eliminated.

Additions & subtractions:

For damp *shao yang* malarial diseases, one-sided foot pain, a heavy, drooping sensation in the arms and legs, more cold and less fever, and a soggy pulse, add Radix Bupleuri (*Chai Hu*), Radix Panacis Ginseng (*Ren Shen*), and Rhizoma Pinelliae Ternatae (*Ban Xia*). This results in *Chai Ping Tang* (Bupleurum Levelling Decoction).

For concomitant heat manifest by a slimy, yellow tongue coating, subtract Licorice and add Rhizoma Coptidis Chinensis (*Huang Lian*).

For damp heat with a bitter taste in the mouth, a dry throat but no thirst, and a yellow, slimy tongue coating, add Radix Scutellariae Baicalensis (*Huang Qin*) and Rhizoma Coptidis Chinensis (*Huang Lian*).

For food stagnation with severe distention and constipation, add Semen Raphani Sativi (*Lai Fu Zi*), Pericarpium Arecae Catechu (*Da Fu Pi*), and Fructus Citri Seu Ponciri (*Zhi Ke*).

Also for food stagnation, add Massa Medica Fermentata (*Shen Qu*), Fructus Germinatus Hordei Vulgaris (*Mai Ya*), and Fructus Crataegi (*Shan Zha*).

For severe epigastric and abdominal distention and fullness, add Radix Saussureae Seu Vladimiriae (*Mu Xiang*) and Fructus Amomi (*Sha Ren*).

For severe vomiting, add Rhizoma Pinelliae Ternatae (*Ban Xia*).

For concomitant exterior pattern with fever and aversion to cold, add Herba Agastachis Seu Pogostemi (*Huo Xiang*), Rhizoma Pinelliae Ternatae (*Ban Xia*), and Folium Perillae Frutescentis (*Su Ye*). This results in *Huo Xiang Zheng Qi San* (Agastachis Righteous Qi Powder).

For severe damp cold with bodily cold and pain, add Cortex Cinnamomi (*Rou Gui*), Fructus Alpiniae Katsumadai (*Cao Dou Kou*), and dry Rhizoma Zingiberis (*Gan Jiang*).

For severe diarrhea, add Rhizoma Atractylodis Macrocephalae (*Bai Zhu*), Sclerotium Poriae Cocos (*Fu Ling*), Semen Plantaginis (*Che Qian Zi*), and Rhizoma Alismatis (*Ze Xie*).

For diarrhea due to stagnation of cold damp evils in the spleen, add *Wu Ling San* (Five *Ling* Powder), *i.e.*, Sclerotium Poriae Cocos (*Fu Ling*), Sclerotium Polypori Umbellati (*Zhu Ling*), Rhizoma Atractylodis Macrocephalae (*Bai Zhu*), Rhizoma Alismatis (*Ze Xie*), and Ramulus Cinnamomi (*Gui Zhi*). This results in *Wei Ling San* (Stomach *Ling* Powder).

For more prominent spleen vacuity with pronounced lack of appetite and fatigue but less distention and fullness, replace Atractylodis with Rhizoma Atractylodis Macrocephalae (*Bai Zhu*) and add Radix

Astragali Membranacei (*Huang Qi*) and Radix Dioscoreae Oppositae (*Shan Yao*).

For cholelithiasis, add Herba Artemisiae Capillaris (*Yin Chen Hao*), Tuber Curcumae (*Yu Jin*), and Fructus Gardeniae Jasminoidis (*Shan Zhi Zi*).

For delayed labor or dead fetus which will not descend, add Mirabilitum (*Mang Xiao*) and Fructus Immaturus Citri Seu Ponciri (*Zhi Shi*).

14.2 *Qing Re Chi Shi Ji* (Heat-clearing, dampness-eliminating formulas)

Representative formulas:

A. *Yin Chen Hao Tang* (Artemisia Capillaris Decoction)

Composition:

Herba Artemisiae Capillaris (*Yin Chen Hao*), 30g
Fructus Gardeniae Jasminoidis (*Zhi Zi*), 15g
Radix Et Rhizoma Rhei (*Da Huang*), 9g, remove the skin

Functions: Clears heat, disinhibits dampness, recedes yellowing

Indications: Damp heat jaundice. Acute hepatitis, hepatic necrosis, cirrhosis, cholecystitis, cholelithiasis, favism, malarial diseases, typhoid fever, leukemia, leptospirosis, nephritis, edema, beriberi, stomatitis, urticaria, pruritus, gingivitis, eye diseases, and uterine bleeding

Main signs & symptoms: Whole body, face, and eyes yellow, the yellow color being bright, slight abdominal fullness, thirst within the mouth, inhibited urination, a slimy, yellow tongue coating, and deep, rapid pulse

Contraindications:

1. Do not use in yin jaundice.
2. Use with caution during pregnancy.

Formula explanation:

In this formula, a heavy dose of Artemisia Capillaris is the sovereign medicinal. It clears and disinhibits dampness and heat as well as recedes jaundice. Gardenia is its minister. It frees and disinhibits the three burners. It conducts damp heat by moving it downward and, thereby, leads out damp heat via the urination. Rhubarb is the assistant. It drains heat and dispels stasis, and frees and disinhibits defecation. These three medicinals combined together discharge downward damp heat, stasis and stagnation and thus automatically recede jaundice.

Additions & subtractions:

For high fever due to severe heat, add Radix Gentianae Scabrae (*Long Dan Cao*), Radix Isatidis Seu Baphicacanthi (*Ban Lan Gen*), and Radix Et Rhizoma Polygoni Cuspidati (*Hu Zhang*).

For serious cases of hepatitis with jaundice, spirit and orientation (*i.e.*, the emotions) befuddled and confused, and a yellow, slimy tongue coating, add Rhizoma Polygoni Cuspidati (*Hu Zhang*) and Rhizoma Acori Graminei (*Shi Chang Pu*).

If there is delirium, add *An Gong Niu Huang Wan* (Quiet the Palace Bezoar Pills); see portal-opening formulas.

For alternating fever and chills with a bitter taste in the mouth, add Radix Bupleuri (*Chai Hu*) and Radix Scutellariae Baicalensis (*Huang Qin*).

Also for fever and chills, add Fructus Forsythiae Suspensae (*Lian Qiao*) and Flos Chrysanthemi Indici (*Ye Ju Hua*).

For hypochondrial and lateral costal pain and abdominal fullness, add Tuber Curcumae (*Yu Jin*) and Fructus Immaturus Citri Seu Ponciri (*Zhi Shi*).

Also for hypochondrial and lateral costal pain, add Radix Bupleuri (*Chai Hu*), Fructus Meliae Toosendan (*Chuan Lian Zi*), Rhizoma Cyperi Rotundi (*Xiang Fu*), and Radix Albus Paeoniae Lactiflorae (*Bai Shao*).

For nausea, vomiting, and indigestion, add Caulis In Taeniis Bambusae (*Zhu Ru*) and Massa Medica Fermentata (*Shen Qu*).

Also for nausea and vomiting, add Caulis In Taeniis Bambusae (*Zhu Ru*) and Folium Eriobotryae Japonicae (*Pi Pa Ye*).

For lack of appetite due to food stagnation, add Massa Medica Fermentata (*Shen Qu*), Fructus Germinatus Hordei Vulgaris (*Mai Ya*), and carbonized Semen Arecae Catechu (*Jiao Bing Lang*).

For cholelithiasis, add Herba Desmodii (*Jin Qian Cao*).

For scanty, reddish yellow urine, add Talcum (*Hua Shi*), Rhizoma Alismatis (*Ze Xie*), and Herba Desmodii (*Jin Qian Cao*).

For difficult and irregular bowel movements, add Herba Eupatorii Fortunei (*Pei Lan*).

B. *Ba Zheng San* (Eight Righteous [Ingredients] Powder)

Composition:

Semen Plantaginis (*Che Qian Zi*), 9g
Herba Dianthi (*Qu Mai*), 9g
Herba Polygoni Avicularis (*Bian Xu*), 9g
Talcum (*Hua Shi*), 15g
Fructus Gardeniae Jasminoidis (*Shan Zhi Zi Ren*), 6g
Radix Glycyrrhizae (*Gan Cao*), 6g, mix-fried
Caulis Akebiae Mutong (*Mu Tong*), 9g
Radix Et Rhizoma Rhei (*Da Huang*), 6g,
Medulla Junci Effusi (*Deng Xin Cao*), 9g

Functions: Clears heat and drains fire, disinhibits water and frees strangury

Indications: Damp heat pouring downward. Acute urinary tract infection, urinary calculi, cystitis, urethritis, acute prostatitis, acute nephritis, acute pyelonephritis, glomerulonephritis, and acute gonorrhea

Main signs & symptoms: Hot strangury, bloody strangury, urination cloudy and red, astringent and painful, dribbling and dripping, uneasy flow, if severe, complete urinary blockage, lower abdominal tension and fullness, a dry mouth and tongue, a slimy, yellow tongue coating, and a slippery, rapid pulse

Contraindications:

1. Do not use long-term since it may cause light-headedness, palpita
   tions, and diminished appetite.
2. Use only with care during pregnancy.
3. Do not use unmodified for vacuity cold.
4. Do not use in persons with bodily vacuity.

Formula explanation:

In this formula, Akebia, Talcum, Plantaginis, Dianthus, and Polygonum Avicularis all disinhibit water and open strangury. They also clear heat and disinhibit dampness. Gardenia clears and drains damp heat from the three burners. Rhubarb discharges heat and downbears fire. Juncus conducts heat and moves it downward. Licorice harmonizes these medicinals and relaxes urgency or tension.

Additions & subtractions:

For bloody urine, add Rhizoma Imperatae Cylindricae (*Bai Mao Gen*), Herba Cephalanoplos (*Xiao Ji*), and Herba Ecliptae Prostratae (*Han Lian Cao*).

Also for painful, bloody urination, increase the dosage of Polygonum Avicularis and add Rhizoma Imperatae Cylindricae (*Bai Mao Gen*) and Herba Cephalanoplos (*Xiao Ji*).

Again for painful, bloody urination, subtract Juncus and add Rhizoma Imperatae Cylindricae (*Mao Gen*).

For stones in the urinary tract, add Spora Lygodii (*Hai Jin Sha*), Herba Desmodii (*Jin Qian Cao*), and Endothelium Corneum Gigeriae Galli (*Ji Nei Jin*).

Also for urinary calculi, add Spora Lygodii (*Hai Jin Sha*), Herba Desmodii (*Jin Qian Cao*), Folium Pyrrosiae (*Shi Wei*), and Radix Achyranthis Bidentatae (*Niu Xi*).

Again for urinary calculi, subtract Juncus and Licorice and add Spora Lygodii (*Hai Jin Sha*) and Herba Desmodii (*Jin Qian Cao*).

For turbid urination, add Rhizoma Dioscoreae Hypoglaucae (*Bi Xie*) and Rhizoma Acori Graminei (*Shi Chang Pu*).

For urinary retention, increase the dosage of Talcum, Polygonum Avicularis, and Akebia and add Cortex Phellodendri (*Huang Bai*) and Cortex Cinnamomi (*Rou Gui*).

Also for urinary retention with a yellow, slimy tongue coating and a rapid, replete pulse due to damp heat evils attacking the bladder, add Succinum (*Hu Po*).

For stomatitis, add Herba Lophatheri Gracilis (*Dan Zhu Ye*) and raw Radix Rehmanniae (*Sheng Di*).

If there is no constipation or there are loose stools, subtract Rhubarb.

C. *Er Miao San* (Two Wonders Powder)

Composition:

Cortex Phellodendri (*Huang Bai*), 9g, stir-fried
Rhizoma Atractylodis (*Cang Zhu*), 12g, soaked in rice-washing water and stir-fried

Functions: Clears heat and dries dampness

Indications: Damp heat leaking through and pouring (down). Lumbago, sacroiliac pain, tinea pedis, eczema, mycotic vaginitis, cervicitis, abnormal vaginal discharge, gonorrhea, urinary tract infection, hepatitis, beriberi, rheumatoid arthritis, gouty arthritis, and gonococcal arthritis

Main signs & symptoms: Sinew and bone aching and pain, damp heat pouring downward, soft atony of both feet with lack of strength, possible redness, swelling, and pain of the feet and knees, possible damp heat vaginal discharge, possible damp ulcers on the lower extremities, short, yellow urination, a slimy, yellow tongue coating, and a soggy, rapid pulse

Contraindications:

1. Do not use unmodified in case of lung heat.
2. Do not use unmodified in case of liver/kidney vacuity.

Formula explanation:

Within this formula, Phellodendron is bitter and cold. Its coldness clears heat and its bitterness dries dampness. It also tends to enter the lower burner. Atractylodis is bitter and warm. It is also able to dry dampness. The combination of these two medicinals clears heat and dries dampness. Once heat is dispelled and dampness is eliminated, all the conditions associated with this pattern are automatically healed.

Additions & subtractions:

For thick, yellow abnormal vaginal discharge, add Semen Euryalis Ferocis (*Qian Shi*), Cortex Cedrelae (*Chun Gen Bai Pi*), and Semen Gingkonis Bilobae (*Bai Guo*).

For severe eczema and itching of the lower part of the body, add Semen Arecae Catechu (*Bing Lang*) and Radix Sophorae Flavescentis (*Ku Shen*).

For weakness and soreness of the low back and knees or burning pain or numbness in the feet, add Radix Achyranthis Bidentatae (*Niu Xi*). This results in *San Miao San* (Three Wonders Powder).

For pain and swelling of the lower limbs, add Radix Achyranthis Bidentatae (*Niu Xi*) and Semen Coicis Lachryma-jobi (*Yi Yi Ren*). This results in *Si Miao San* (Four Wonders Powder).

For atony and lack of strength of the lower extremities with possible slight edema and numbness and a sensation of heat which begins on the dorsum of the foot and proceeds up the legs to the waist, add

206

Radix Cyathulae (*Chuan Niu Xi*), Radix Angelicae Sinensis (*Dang Gui Wei*), Radix Stephaniae Tetrandrae (*Han Fan Ji*), Rhizoma Dioscoreae Hypoglaucae (*Bi Xie*), and mix-fried Radix Glycyrrhizae (*Zhi Gan Cao*). This results in *Jia Wei Er Miao San* (Added Flavors Two Wonders Powder).

For tinea pedis, add Semen Coicis Lachryma-jobi (*Yi Yi Ren*), Fructus Chaenomelis Lagenariae (*Mu Gua*), and Semen Arecae Catechu (*Bing Lang*).

For beriberi with scanty, reddish urination, and a red tongue with yellow, slimy coating, add Semen Arecae Catechu (*Bing Lang*).

14.3 *Li Shui Shen Shi Ji* (Water-disinhibiting, dampness-percolating formulas)

Representative formula: *Wu Ling San* (Five *Ling* Powder)

Composition:

Sclerotium Polypori Umbellati (*Zhu Ling*), 9g
Rhizoma Alismatis (*Ze Xie*), 15g
Rhizoma Atractylodis Macrocephalae (*Bai Zhu*), 9g
Sclerotium Poriae Cocos (*Fu Ling*), 9g
Ramulus Cinnamomi (*Gui Zhi*), 6g, remove the bark

Functions: Disinhibit water and percolate dampness, warm yang and transform qi

Indications: 1) Exterior pattern with interior stoppage of water dampness, 2) water dampness stopped internally, and 3) Phlegm rheum. Chronic nephritic edema, acute and chronic nephritis, chronic renal failure, acute gastritis, cardiac edema from congestive heart failure, gastroptosis, gastrectasis, ascites due to liver cirrhosis, infectious hepatitis, urinary retention, scrotal hydrocele, acute gastroenteritis with diarrhea, Meniere's disease, genitourinary tract infections, and neurogenic bladder syndrome

Main signs & symptoms: 1) Headache, fever, vexatious thirst, desire to drink but vomiting upon entering of water (into the stomach), inhibited urination, a white tongue coating with a floating pulse; 2) edema, diarrhea, inhibited urination, cholera-like vomiting and diarrhea patterns; and 3) throbbing palpitations below the umbilicus, vomiting frothy saliva and vertigo or shortness of breath and coughing

Contraindications:

1. Do not use or overuse in patients with spleen and kidney vacuity or combine with medicinals which supplement and nourish the spleen and stomach and supplement and enrich the kidneys.
2. Do not use for the treatment of yin vacuity dysuria.
3. Do not use for prolonged periods of time.

Formula explanation:

Within this formula, relatively heavy doses of Alisma are used as the sovereign medicinal. Alisma is sweet, bland, and percolating, while its nature is cold. It out-thrusts the bladder, disinhibits water, and percolates dampness. The minister medicinals are Poria and Polyporus which also blandly percolate. They help strengthen the disinhibition of water. Added to these is Atractylodis which fortifies spleen qi and transports and transforms water dampness. The assistant medicinal is Cinnamon which is a single medicinal with two uses. First, externally, it resolves the *tai yang* on the exterior. Secondly, it aids bladder qi internally. When these five medicinals are combined together, water is moved and qi is transformed, the exterior is relieved and the spleen in fortified.

Additions & subtractions:

If the qi is simultaneously vacuous, add Radix Astragali Membranacei (*Huang Qi*).

If yang is simultaneously vacuous, add Radix Praeparatus Aconiti Carmichaeli (*Fu Zi*).

If there is pronounced edema, increase the dosages of all ingredients or add Semen Plantaginis (*Che Qian Zi*).

For serious edema, add Radix Astragali Membranacei (*Huang Qi*) and Radix Stephaniae Tetrandrae (*Han Fang Ji*).

Also for serious edema, add Cortex Radicis Mori (*Sang Bai Pi*), Pericarpium Arecae Catechu (*Da Fu Pi*), and Pericarpium Citri Reticulatae (*Chen Pi*).

For cold damp painful *bi* with thirst and urinary difficulty, add Radix Et Rhizoma Notopterygii (*Qiang Huo*).

For serious exterior patterns, add Herba Ephedrae (*Ma Huang*) and Folium Perillae Frutescentis (*Su Ye*).

For diarrhea and decreased urination, subtract Cinnamon. This results in *Si Ling San* (Four *Ling* Powder).

For vomiting, diarrhea, and abdominal distention, add Rhizoma Atractylodis (*Cang Zhu*), Cortex Magnoliae Officinalis (*Hou Po*), and Pericarpium Citri Reticulatae (*Ju Pi*).

For damp heat diarrhea, subtract Atractylodis and Cinnamon and add Herba Artemisiae Capillaris (*Yin Chen Hao*) and Flos Lonicerae Japonicae (*Jin Yin Hua*).

For jaundice with dysuria, add Herba Artemisiae Capillaris (*Yin Chen Hao*). This results in *Yin Chen Wu Ling San* (Artemisia Five *Ling* Powder).

Also for jaundice and dysuria, to the above add Fructus Gardeniae Jasminoidis (*Shan Zhi Zi*).

For edema with concomitant qi stagnation, add *Wu Pi Yin* (Five Peels Drink), *i.e.*, Cortex Sclerotii Poriae Cocos (*Fu Ling Pi*), Cortex Radicis Mori (*Sang Bai Pi*), Cortex Rhizomatis Zingiberis (*Sheng Jiang Pi*), Pericarpium Arecae Catechu (*Da Fu Pi*), and Pericarpium Citri Reticulatae (*Chen Pi*).

For liver/spleen disharmony and for *shao yang* division patterns, add *Xiao Chai Hu Tang* (Minor Bupleurum Decoction), *i.e.*, Radix Bupleuri (*Chai Hu*), Radix Scutellariae Baicalensis (*Huang Qin*), Radix Codonopsis Pilosulae (*Dang Shen*), Rhizoma Pinelliae Ternatae (*Ban Xia*), mix-fried Radix Glycyrrhizae (*Zhi Gan Cao*), Fructus Zizyphi Jujubae (*Da Zao*), and raw Rhizoma Zingiberis (*Sheng Jiang*). This results in *Chai Ling Tang* (Bupleurum & *Ling* Decoction).

For hematuria and burning pain, add Talcum (*Hua Shi*) and Gelatinum Corii Asini (*E Jiao*).

For joint pain and generalized edema but especially of the lower extremities, add Radix Ledebouriellae Sesloidis (*Fang Feng*), Radix Et Rhizoma Notopterygii (*Qiang Huo*), and Radix Codonopsis Pilosulae (*Dang Shen*).

For heart palpitations, insomnia, or gastric ulcer, add Radix Saussureae Seu Vladimiriae (*Mu Xiang*), Rhizoma Coptidis Chinensis (*Huang Lian*), and raw Rhizoma Zingiberis (*Sheng Jiang*).

14.4 *Wen Hua Shui Shi Ji* (Warming & transforming water dampness formulas)

Representative formula: *Ling Gui Zhu Gan Tang* (Poria, Cinnamon, Atractylodis, & Licorice Decoction)

Composition:

Sclerotium Poriae Cocos (*Fu Ling*), 12g
Ramulus Cinnamomi (*Gui Zhi*), 9g
Rhizoma Atractylodis Macrocephalae (*Bai Zhu*), 6g
Radix Glycyrrhizae (*Gan Cao*), 6g, mix-fried

Functions: Warms and transforms phlegm rheum, fortifies the spleen and disinhibits dampness

Indications: Central yang insufficiency phlegm rheum disease. Chronic bronchitis, bronchial asthma, pulmonary emphysema, cardiac or nephrotic edema, valvular disease, Basedow's disease, Meniere's disease, neurosis, neurasthenia, hysteria, motion sickness, rheumatoid arthritis, chronic gastritis, chronic nephritis, renal atrophy, hypertension, sinusitis, rhinitis, anemia, conjunctivitis, chronic optic nerve disorders, optic nerve atrophy, and nebula

Main signs & symptoms: Chest and lateral costal propping fullness, vertigo, heart palpitations, possible shortness of breath and coughing, a white, slimy tongue coating, and a wiry, slippery or deep, tight pulse

Formula explanation:

Within this formula, Poria is the sovereign. It fortifies the spleen and percolates dampness, dispels phlegm and transforms rheum. Cinnamon is the minister. It warms yang and transforms qi. When yang is warmed, rheum is transformed. It is also able to transform the qi in order to disinhibit water. Simultaneously, it levels (up-)thrusting and downbears counterflow. Combined with Poria, one warms and one disinhibits. Thus water rheum stagnation and retention categorized as cold is warmed, transformed, percolated, and disinhibited. The origin of dampness is the spleen. If there is spleen vacuity, this engenders dampness. Therefore, Atractylodis is used as an assistant to fortify the spleen and dry dampness, thus aiding spleen transportation and transformation. Once spleen yang is fortified and effulgent, water dampness is cured automatically. The messenger is Licorice which boosts the qi and harmonizes the center.

Additions & subtractions:

For edema, add Radix Astragali Membranacei (*Huang Qi*) Radix Stephaniae Tetrandrae (*Fang Ji*), and Rhizoma Alismatis (*Ze Xie*).

For excessive phlegm, add Fructus Perillae Frutescentis (*Su Zi*), Semen Lepedii (*Ting Li Zi*), and Fructus Zizyphi Jujubae (*Da Zao*).

For vomiting watery fluids and phlegm, add Rhizoma Pinelliae Ternatae (*Ban Xia*) and Pericarpium Citri Reticulatae (*Chen Pi*).

For severe vomiting and belching, add Calyx Diospyros Kaki (*Shi Di*) and Fructus Amomi (*Sha Ren*).

For glomus and pain in the epigastrium, add Fructus Citri Seu Ponciri (*Zhi Ke*) and Cortex Magnoliae Officinalis (*Hou Po*).

For Meniere's disease, add *Zhen Wu Tang* (True Warrior's Decoction), *i.e.*, Radix Praeparatus Aconiti Carmichaeli (*Fu Zi*), Rhizoma Atractylodis Macrocephalae (*Bai Zhu*), Sclerotium Poriae Cocos (*Fu Ling*), Radix Albus Paeoniae Lactiflorae (*Bai Shao*), and raw Rhizoma Zingiberis (*Sheng Jiang*).

If spleen qi vacuity is severe with fatigue and lethargy, add Radix Codonopsis Pilosulae (*Dang Shen*).

14.5 *Chu Feng Sheng Shi Ji* (Dispelling wind, overcoming dampness formulas)

Representative formula: *Du Huo Ji Sheng Tang* (*Du Huo & Loranthus Decoction*)

Composition:

Radix Angelicae Pubescentis (*Du Huo*), 9g
Ramus Loranthi Seu Visci (*Ji Sheng*), 6g
Cortex Eucommiae Ulmoidis (*Du Zhong*), 6g
Radix Achyranthis Bidentatae (*Niu Xi*), 6g
Herba Cum Radice Asari (*Xi Xin*), 6g
Radix Gentianae Macrophyllae (*Qin Jiao*), 6g
Sclerotium Poriae Cocos (*Fu Ling*), 6g
Cortex Cinnamomi (*Rou Gui Xin*), 6g
Radix Ledebouriellae Sesloidis (*Fang Feng*), 6g
Rhizoma Ligustici Wallichii (*Chuan Xiong*), 6g
Radix Panacis Ginseng (*Ren Shen*), 6g
Radix Glycyrrhizae (*Gan Cao*), 6g
Radix Angelicae Sinensis (*Dang Gui*), 6g
Radix Albus Paeoniae Lactiflorae (*Bai Shao*), 6g
dry Radix Rehmanniae (*Gan Di Huang*), 6g

Functions: Dispels wind dampness, stops *bi* pain, boosts the liver and kidneys, supplements the qi and blood

Indications: Chronic *bi* patterns, liver/kidney dual deficiency, qi and blood insufficiency. Chronic rheumatoid arthritis, osteoarthritis, rheumatic sciatica, lumbar strain, lumbar intervertebral disc herniation, pain in the midline and back during pregnancy, hemiplegia due to stroke, and the sequelae of poliomyelitis

Main signs & symptoms: Low back and knee aching and pain, inhibition of the joints of the limbs, possible numbness and loss of feeling, intolerance to cold and liking warmth, palpitations, shortness of breath, a pale tongue with white coating, and a fine, weak pulse

Contraindications:

1. Do not use for acute arthritis.

Formula explanation:

In this formula, *Du Huo* is the sovereign. It rectifies hidden wind and dispels wind, cold, damp evils from the lower burner and sinews and bones. Asarum emits and scatters wind cold from the yin channels and sweeps away wind dampness from out of the sinews and bones, thus stopping pain. Ledebouriella dispels wind evils and overcomes dampness. Gentiana Macrophylla eliminates wind dampness and relaxes the sinews. Loranthus, Eucommia, and Achyranthis dispel wind dampness while simultaneously supplementing the liver and kidneys. *Dang Gui*, Ligusticum, Rehmannia, and Peony nourish the blood while simultaneously quickening the blood. Ginseng and Poria supplement the qi and fortify the spleen. Cinnamon warms and opens the blood vessels, and Licorice regulates and harmonizes all these other medicinals. Thus this prescription as a whole dispels evils and supports the righteous.

Additions & subtractions:

For severe cold, add Radix Praeparatus Aconiti Carmichaeli (*Fu Zi*) and dry Rhizoma Zingiberis (*Gan Jiang*).

For severe dampness, add Radix Stephaniae Tetrandrae (*Fang Ji*) and Rhizoma Atractylodis (*Cang Zhu*).

For severe pain, add Lumbricus (*Di Long*), Agkistrodon Seu Bungarus Multinetus (*Bai Hua She*), and Flos Carthami Tinctorii (*Hong Hua*).

Also for severe pain, add Radix Aconiti (*Chuan Wu Tou*).

For blood stasis, add Semen Pruni Persicae (*Tao Ren*) and Flos Carthami Tinctorii (*Hong Hua*).

If vacuity is mild, subtract Ginseng, Rehmannia, and Peony.

For the sequelae of poliomyelitis, add Radix Pseudoginseng (*San Qi*), Radix Clematidis (*Wei Ling Xian*), and Fructus Chaenomelis Lagenariae (*Mu Gua*).

桑菊飲中桔梗翹
杏仁甘草薄荷饒
蘆根爲引輕清劑
熱盛陽明入母膏

Mnemonic verse for learning *Sang Ju Yin*

15

Zhu Tan Ji
Dispelling Phlegm Formulas

Phlegm is a yin evil. It is congealed from body fluids and water dampness. Body fluids are transported and transformed by qi. If qi becomes insufficient or depressed, fluids and humors may not be transported and transformed properly. In that case, they may gather and accumulate, eventually congealing into phlegm. It is also possible for heat and fire to steam the juices and congeal body fluids into phlegm. Once generated, phlegm itself may hinder and obstruct the free flow of qi, blood, and body fluids. Depending upon its cause and the patient's bodily constitution, phlegm may be either hot or cold, damp or dry, and may exist either under the skin, in the channels and network vessels, or in the viscera.

There are five subcategories of phlegm-dispelling formulas. These are: 1) Formulas which dry dampness and transform phlegm. These fortify the spleen and transform phlegm and are used to treat cough with phlegm dampness. 2) Formulas which clear heat and transform phlegm. These are used to treat hot phlegm patterns. 3) Formulas which moisten dryness and transform phlegm. These are used to treat dry phlegm patterns. 4) Formulas which warm and transform cold phlegm. These warm the lungs and transform phlegm and are typically used to treat phlegm due to spleen yang vacuity or phlegm rheum obstructing the lungs patterns. 5) Formulas which treat wind and transform phlegm. These are used to treat either external wind invading the lungs resulting in phlegm accumulation or retention of turbid phlegm with internal stirring of liver wind.

15.1 *Zao Shi Hua Tan Ji* (Drying dampness, transforming phlegm formulas)

Representative formula: *Er Chen Tang* (Two Aged [Ingredients] Decoction)

Composition:

Rhizoma Pinelliae Ternatae (*Ban Xia*), 15g
Pericarpium Citri Reticulatae (*Ju Pi*), 15g
Sclerotium Poriae Cocos (*Bai Fu Ling*), 9g
Radix Glycyrrhizae (*Gan Cao*), 5g, mix-fried
raw Rhizoma Zingiberis (*Sheng Jiang*), 7 slices
Fructus Pruni Wumei (*Wu Mei*), 1 whole one

Functions: Dries dampness and transforms phlegm, rectifies the qi and harmonizes the center

Indications: Damp phlegm cough. Chronic tracheitis, chronic bronchitis, pulmonary emphysema, goiter, chronic gastritis, peptic ulcer, eclampsia, hangover, gastroptosis, Meniere's disease, and neurosis

Main signs & symptoms: Excessive phlegm which is colored white and easily spit out, chest and diaphragm glomus and oppression, nausea and vomiting, fatigue of the body and limbs, possible vertigo and palpitations, a white, moist tongue coating, and a slippery pulse

Contraindications:

1. Do not use unmodified for lung yin vacuity cough.

Formula explanation:

In this formula, Pinellia is the sovereign. It is acrid and warm and its nature is drying. It is able to dry dampness and transform phlegm as well as to downbear counterflow and harmonize the stomach and thus stop vomiting. Orange Peel is the minister. It rectifies the qi and dries dampness. It aids in normalizing the qi and dispersing phlegm. The assistants are Poria, fresh Ginger, and Mume. Poria fortifies the spleen and percolates dampness. Once dampness is removed, the spleen may become effulgent and phlegm can no longer be engendered. Fresh Ginger downbears counterflow and transforms rheum. It is also able to control the toxins in Pinellia. It also helps Pinellia and Orange Peel move the qi and disperse phlegm. A small amount of Mume is used to restrain the lung qi. Combined with Pinellia, these two scatter and restrain at the same time. Thus phlegm is dispelled without damaging the righteous. Licorice is the messenger. It regulates and harmonizes all these other medicinals. Simultaneously it moistens the lungs and harmonizes center.

Additions & subtractions:

For hot phlegm with irritability, timidity, insomnia, and palpitations, subtract Ginger and Mume and add Caulis In Taeniis Bambusae (*Zhu Ru*), Fructus Immaturus Citri Seu Ponciri (*Zhi Shi*), and Fructus Zizyphi Jujubae (*Da Zao*). This results in *Wen Dan Tang* (Warm the Gallbladder Decoction).

If vexatious heat is more severe, to the above add Rhizoma Coptidis Chinensis (*Huang Lian*). This results in *Huang Lian Wen Dan Tang* (Coptis Warm the Gallbladder Decoction).

For wind stroke with phlegm veiling the portals of the heart, to the above add bile(-treated) Rhizoma Arisaematis (*Dan Xing*), Radix Panacis Ginseng (*Ren Shen*), and Rhizoma Acori Graminei (*Chang Pu*). This results in *Di Tan Tang* (Flush Phlegm Decoction).

219

For common cold with profuse phlegm in the elderly complicated by lung/kidney vacuity, add Radix Angelicae Sinensis (*Dang Gui*) and prepared Radix Rehmanniae (*Shu Di*). This results in *Jin Shui Liu Jun Jian* (Metal & Water Six Gentleman Decoction).

For vomiting due to stomach cold, add Radix Saussureae Seu Vladimiriae (*Mu Xiang*) and Fructus Amomi (*Sha Ren*). This results in *Xiang Sha Er Chen Tang* (Saussurea & Amomum Two Aged [Ingredients] Decoction).

For cold phlegm, add dry Rhizoma Zingiberis (*Gan Jiang*) and Herba Cum Radice Asari (*Xi Xin*).

For hot phlegm, add Radix Scutellariae Baicalensis (*Huang Qin*), Semen Trichosanthis Kirlowii (*Gua Lou Ren*), and Herba Houttuyniae Cordatae (*Yu Xing Cao*).

Also for hot phlegm, add Fructus Trichosanthis Kirlowii (*Gua Lou*) and Concretio Silicea Bambusae (*Tian Zhu Huang*).

For wind phlegm, add bile(-treated) Rhizoma Arisaematis (*Dan Xing*) and Rhizoma Typhonii Gigantaeae (*Bai Fu Zi*).

For phlegm complicated by food stagnation, add Semen Raphani Sativi (*Lai Fu Zi*).

For severe distention and fullness in the chest and diaphragm, add Caulis Perillae Frutescentis (*Su Geng*), Fructus Citri Seu Ponciri (*Zhi Ke*), and Caulis Agastachis (*Huo Geng*).

For indigestion due to food stagnation, add Semen Raphani Sativi (*Lai Fu Zi*) and Massa Medica Fermentata (*Shen Qu*).

For poor appetite and loose stools, subtract Mume and add Radix Panacis Ginseng (*Ren Shen*) and Rhizoma Atractylodis Macrocephalae (*Bai Zhu*).

For ulcers and gastric distress, add Cortex Magnoliae Officinalis (*Hou Po*), Rhizoma Atractylodis (*Cang Zhu*), and Fructus Zizyphi Jujubae (*Da Zao*).

Also for ulcers with a combination of cold and heat, add Cortex Magnoliae Officinalis (*Hou Po*), Radix Panacis Ginseng (*Ren Shen*), Cortex Cinnamomi (*Rou Gui*), and Radix Scutellariae Baicalensis (*Huang Qin*).

For headache and dizziness and, in severe cases, phlegm inversion (*i.e.*, unconsciousness) with cough, nausea, chest and diaphragm glomus and obstruction, vomiting, and reduced appetite complicated by liver wind, subtract Mume and add Rhizoma Arisaematis (*Nan Xing*) and Fructus Immaturus Citri Seu Ponciri (*Zhi Shi*). This results in *Dao Tan Tang* (Lead Out Phlegm Decoction).

For severe dizziness, add Rhizoma Gastrodiae (*Tian Ma*).

For damp heat in the upper burner, add Radix Scutellariae Baicalensis (*Huang Qin*), Fructus Gardeniae Jasminoidis (*Shan Zhi*), Semen Pruni Armeniacae (*Xing Ren*), and Radix Platycodi Grandiflori (*Jie Geng*).

For damp heat in the middle burner, add Herba Agastachis Seu Pogostemi (*Huo Xiang*), Rhizoma Coptidis Chinensis (*Huang Lian*), Cortex Magnoliae Officinalis (*Hou Po*), and Semen Coicis Lachryma-jobi (*Yi Yi Ren*).

For damp heat in the lower burner, add Radix Sophorae Flavescentis (*Ku Shen*), Cortex Phellodendri (*Huang Bai*), and Talcum (*Hua Shi*).

221

For wind dampness, add Radix Clematidis (*Wei Ling Xian*), Radix Gentianae Macrophyllae (*Qin Jiao*), Fructus Xanthii (*Cang Er Zi*), and Ramulus Cinnamomi (*Gui Zhi*).

For exterior patterns with aversion to cold and fever, add Folium Perillae Frutescentis (*Su Ye*), Semen Pruni Armeniacae (*Xing Ren*), and Radix Platycodi Grandiflori (*Jie Geng*).

For cough with profuse phlegm due to external invasion by wind cold, add Herba Ephedrae (*Ma Huang*) and Semen Pruni Armeniacae (*Xing Ren*).

For vomiting of clear fluids, add Rhizoma Atractylodis (*Cang Zhu*) and Rhizoma Atractylodis Macrocephalae (*Bai Zhu*).

For sudden chaos (*i.e.*, cholera-like diseases) with vomiting and diarrhea, add Radix Panacis Ginseng (*Ren Shen*), Radix Praeparatus Aconiti Carmichaeli (*Fu Zi*), Rhizoma Coptidis Chinensis (*Huang Lian*), and Fructus Zizyphi Jujubae (*Da Zao*).

For long-standing phlegm in the channels and muscles with rubbery nodulation, add Concha Ostreae (*Mu Li*), Radix Scrophulariae Ningpoensis (*Xuan Shen*), Thallus Algae (*Kun Bu*), and Herba Sargassii (*Hai Zao*).

For spleen/kidney yang vacuity with cough accompanied by thin, watery phlegm, a deep pulse, and astringent urination, add Cortex Cinnamomi (*Rou Gui*) and Radix Praeparatus Aconiti Carmichaeli (*Fu Zi*).

For insomnia at night but lethargy during the day which becomes worse after meals, add Rhizoma Atractylodis Macrocephalae (*Bai Zhu*) and Rhizoma Acori Graminei (*Chang Pu*).

For severe coughing at night due to a combination of phlegm and blood vacuity, add Radix Angelicae Sinensis (*Dang Gui*).

For damp phlegm obstructing the uterus with menstrual irregularity and copious abnormal vaginal discharge, add Rhizoma Ligustici Wallichii (*Chuan Xiong*) and Radix Angelicae Sinensis (*Dang Gui*).

If there is concomitant dryness, subtract Pinellia and add Fructus Trichosanthis Kirlowii (*Gua Lou*) and Bulbus Fritillariae Cirrhosae (*Chuan Bei Mu*).

For plum pit qi and nausea during pregnancy, add Cortex Magnoliae Officinalis (*Hou Po*) and Folium Perillae Frutescentis (*Su Ye*).

For food-poisoning and summerheat patterns, add Rhizoma Atractylodis (*Cang Zhu*), Cortex Magnoliae Officinalis (*Hou Po*), Herba Agastachis Seu Pogostemi (*Huo Xiang*), and Fructus Zizyphi Jujubae (*Da Zao*).

15.2 *Qing Re Hua Tan Ji* (Heat-clearing, phlegm-transforming formulas)

Representative formula: *Qing Qi Hua Tan Wan* (Clear the Qi, Transform Phlegm Pills)

Composition:

Semen Trichosanthis Kirlowii (*Gua Lou Ren*), 9g
Pericarpium Citri Reticulatae (*Chen Pi*), 6g, remove the white
Radix Scutellariae Baicalensis (*Huang Qin*), 6g, wine-fried
Semen Pruni Armeniacae (*Xing Ren*), 9g, remove the skin and tip
Fructus Immaturus Citri Seu Ponciri (*Zhi Shi*), 6g, stir-fried
Sclerotium Poriae Cocos (*Fu Ling*), 12g
bile(-treated) Rhizoma Arisaematis (*Dan Nan Xing*), 3g

processed Rhizoma Pinelliae Ternatae (*Zhi Ban Xia*), 6g

Functions: Clears heat and transforms phlegm, rectifies the qi and stops coughing

Indications: Phlegm heat internally binding. Chronic tracheitis, acute and chronic bronchitis, bronchiectasis, pneumonia, chronic rhinitis, and nasosinusitis

Main signs & symptoms: Cough with yellow phlegm which is thick and difficult to expectorate, chest and diaphragm glomus and fullness, urination short and reddish, a red tongue with a slimy, yellow coating, and a slippery, rapid pulse

Formula explanation:

Bile-treated Arisaema is the sovereign medicinal in this formula. Its flavor is bitter and its nature is cold. It clears heat and transforms phlegm and it treats replete phlegm and replete fire obstruction and blockage. Scutellaria and Semen Trichosanthis are the minister medicinals. They downbear lung fire and transform hot phlegm. They assist the power of Arisaema. Because the treatment of phlegm also requires the rectification of the qi, Citrus Immaturus and Orange Peel descend the qi and open glomus, disperse phlegm and scatter nodulation. Poria is one of the assistants. It fortifies the spleen and percolates dampness. Armeniaca is another assistant. It diffuses and disinhibits the lung qi. Pinellia is the third assistant. It dries dampness and transforms phlegm. When all these medicinals are combined together, they cleat heat and transform phlegm, rectify the qi and stop coughing. Once heat is cleared and fire downborne, qi normalized and phlegm dispersed, all pathological conditions associated with this pattern are automatically resolved.

Additions & subtractions:

For intense heat in the lungs, add Gypsum (*Shi Gao*) and Rhizoma Anemarrhenae (*Zhi Mu*).

Also for intense heat, subtract Pinellia and add Gypsum (*Shi Gao*).

For dry stools and constipation, add Radix Et Rhizoma Rhei (*Da Huang*).

Also for constipation, add Rhizoma Polygoni Cuspidati (*Hu Zhang*).

For copious yellow and green phlegm, add Herba Houttuyniae Cordatae (*Yu Xing Cao*) and Radix Trichosanthis Kirlowii (*Tian Hua Fen*).

For sticky, tenacious phlegm, subtract Pinellia and add Semen Benincasae Hispidae (*Dong Gua Ren*).

15.3 *Ru Zao Hua Tan Ji* (Dryness-moistening, phlegm-transforming formulas)

Representative formula: *Bei Mu Gua Lou San* (Fritillaria & Trichosanthis Powder)

Composition:

Bulbus Fritillariae (*Bei Mu*), 9g
Fructus Trichosanthis Kirlowii (*Gua Lou*),12g
Radix Trichosanthis Kirlowii (*Tian Hua Fen*), 12g
Sclerotium Poriae Cocos (*Fu Ling*), 9g
Exocarpium Citri Rubri (*Ju Hong*), 6g
Radix Platycodi Grandiflori (*Jie Geng*), 9g

Functions: Moistens the lungs and clears heat, rectifies the qi and transforms phlegm

Indications: Lung dryness with phlegm. Sore throat, bronchitis, tracheitis, laryngitis, pulmonary emphysema, cervical lymphadenitis, thyroiditis, and diabetes mellitus with polydipsia and polyuria

Main signs & symptoms: Tenacious phlegm which is astringent and difficult to spit up, cough, dry throat, a red, dry tongue with scant coating, and a rapid pulse

Contraindications:

1. Do not use for cough with lung yin vacuity.

Formula explanation:

Fritillaria is the sovereign medicinal within this formula. It clears heat and moistens the lungs, transforms phlegm and stops cough. It also opens phlegm qi depression binding. Fructus Trichosanthis is the minister. It clears heat and moistens dryness, rectifies the qi and washes away phlegm. It also opens *bi* and obstruction in the chest and diaphragm. Radix Trichosanthis clears heat and transforms phlegm, generates fluids and moistens dryness. Poria fortifies the spleen and disinhibits dampness, remembering that the spleen is the origin of phlegm generation. Red Orange Peel rectifies the qi and transforms phlegm, thus assisting in normalizing the qi and dispersing phlegm. Platycodon diffuses and disinhibits the lung qi, thus reestablishing lung metal's authority over diffusing and downbearing. Therefore, by using these medicinals in combination, lung dryness is moistened and phlegm is automatically transformed; clearing and depurating are restored and coughing is automatically stopped.

Additions & subtractions:

For severe dry, sore throat, add Tuber Ophiopogonis Japonicae (*Mai Dong*), Radix Scrophulariae Ningpoensis (*Xuan Shen*), and Radix Glycyrrhizae (*Gan Cao*).

Also for severe dry, sore throat, add Tuber Ophiopogonis Japonicae (*Mai Dong*), Radix Scrophulariae Ningpoensis (*Xuan Shen*), and Rhizoma Anemarrhenae (*Zhi Mu*).

For cough with a ticklish sensation in the throat, add Radix Peucedani (*Qian Hu*) and Fructus Arctii Lappae (*Niu Bang Zi*).

For hoarseness and blood-streaked phlegm, subtract Red Orange Peel and add Radix Glehniae Littoralis (*Sha Shen*) and Gelatinum Corii Asini (*E Jiao*).

Also for bloody phlegm, add Gelatinum Corii Asini (*E Jiao*), Herba Ecliptae Prostratae (*Han Lian Cao*), and raw Radix Rehmanniae (*Sheng Di*).

Again for bloody phlegm, subtract Red Orange Peel and add Radix Glehniae Littoralis (*Sha Shen*), Tuber Ophiopogonis Japonicae (*Mai Dong*), Rhizoma Phragmitis Communis (*Lu Gen*), and Herba Agrimoniae Pilosae (*Xian He Cao*).

For severe coughing and wheezing, add Semen Pruni Armeniacae (*Xing Ren*), Folium Eriobotryae Japonicae (*Pi Pa Ye*), and Flos Tussilaginis Farfarae (*Kuan Dong Hua*).

For concomitant exterior pattern, add Folium Mori Albi (*Sang Bai Ye*), Semen Pruni Armeniacae (*Xing Ren*), Radix Peucedani (*Qian Hu*), and Fructus Arctii Lappae (*Niu Bang Zi*).

For diabetes mellitus, increase the dosage of Radix Trichosanthis.

Comment: This condition should be treated by a combination of dryness-moistening and phlegm-transforming medicinals and should not be mistaken for lung yin vacuity, in which case, greasy, yin-enriching ingredients may aggravate phlegm by damaging the spleen and inhibiting the qi.

15.4 *Wen Hua Han Tan Ji* (Warming & transforming cold phlegm formulas)

Representative formula: *Ling Gan Wu Wei Jiang Xi Tang* (Poria, Licorice, Schizandra, Ginger, & Asarum Decoction)

Composition:

Sclerotium Poriae Cocos (*Fu Ling*), 12g
Radix Glycyrrhizae (*Gan Cao*), 6g
dry Rhizoma Zingiberis (*Gan Jiang*), 9g
Herba Cum Radice Asari (*Xi Xin*), 6g
Fructus Schizandrae Chinensis (*Wu Wei Zi*), 6g

Functions: Warms the lungs and transforms rheum

Indications: Cold rheum internally amassed. Chronic tracheitis, acute and chronic bronchitis, bronchial asthma, pulmonary emphysema, chronic pulmonary obstructive disease, edema, ascites, chronic nephritis, atrophic kidney, pleurisy, beriberi, and cardiac asthma

Main signs & symptoms: Cough with copious phlegm which is clear, watery, and white in color, chest and diaphragm not well, a white, slimy tongue coating, and a wiry, slippery pulse

Formula explanation:

Dry Ginger is the sovereign medicinal in this formula. It is acrid and its nature is hot. Therefore, it warms the lungs and scatters cold, thus transforming phlegm. It also warms and transports spleen yang, thus dispelling dampness. Asarum is the minister. It also is acrid and scattering. Asarum warms the lungs and scatters cold and assists dry Ginger in scattering congelation and gathering of rheum. Poria is another minister. It is sweet and bland. Poria fortifies the spleen and percolates dampness. Thus one minister transforms gatherings of phlegm and one addresses the source of phlegm generation. The assistant is Schizandra which restrains lung qi and stops cough. Combined with Asarum, one scatters and one restrains. Thus there is scattering without damaging the righteous and there is restraining without retaining evils. The messenger is Licorice. It harmonizes the center as well as regulates and harmonizes all the other medicinals.

Additions & subtractions:

If there is copious phlegm and a desire to vomit, add Rhizoma Pinelliae Ternatae (*Ban Xia*) to downbear counterflow and stop vomiting, dry dampness and transform phlegm.

If there is simultaneous thrusting qi counterflowing above, add Ramulus Cinnamomi (*Gui Zhi*) to warm the center and downbear counterflow.

If cough is severe and there is facial edema, add Semen Pruni Armeniacae (*Xing Ren*), Flos Tussilaginis Farfarae (*Kuan Dong Hua*), and Radix Asteris Tartarici (*Zi Wan*) to diffuse and disinhibit lung qi and stop coughing.

For chest and epigastric distention and fullness, add Pericarpium Citri Reticulatae (*Chen Pi*) and Fructus Amomi (*Sha Ren*).

Also for chest and epigastric distention and fullness, add Fructus Citri Seu Ponciri (*Zhi Ke*) and Pericarpium Citri Reticulatae (*Ju Pi*).

For loss of appetite and fatigue due to spleen qi vacuity, add Radix Codonopsis Pilosulae (*Dang Shen*) and Rhizoma Atractylodis Macrocephalae (*Bai Zhu*).

Also for loss of appetite, add Rhizoma Atractylodis Macrocephalae (*Bai Zhu*) and Radix Dioscoreae Oppositae (*Shan Yao*).

For patients with bodily vacuity, add Cordyceps Sinensis (*Dong Chong Xia Cao*).

For aversion to cold and fever, add Folium Perillae Frutescentis (*Su Ye*) and Radix Platycodi Grandiflori (*Jie Geng*).

For wheezing and dyspnea, add Herba Ephedrae (*Ma Huang*) and Semen Pruni Armeniacae (*Xing Ren*).

15.5 *Zhi Feng Hua Tan Ji* (Wind-treating, phlegm-transforming formulas)

Representative formula: *Ban Xia Bai Zhu Tian Ma Tang* (Pinellia, Atractylodes, & Gastrodia Decoction)

Composition:

Rhizoma Pinelliae Ternatae (*Ban Xia*), 9g
Rhizoma Gastrodiae Elatae (*Tian Ma*), 6g
Sclerotium Poriae Cocos (*Fu Ling*), 6g
Exocarpium Citri Rubri (*Ju Hong*), 6g
Rhizoma Atractylodis Macrocephalae (*Bai Zhu*), 15g
Radix Glycyrrhizae (*Gan Cao*), 4g
raw Rhizoma Zingiberis (*Sheng Jiang*), 1 slice

Fructus Zizyphi Jujubae (*Da Zao*), 2 pieces

Functions: Dries dampness and transforms phlegm, levels the liver and extinguishes wind

Indications: Wind and phlegm harassing above. Recurrent headaches and dizziness, Meniere's disease, neurotic vertigo, hypertension, tubercular meningitis, and orthostatic hypotension

Main signs & symptoms: Dizziness, vertigo, headache, chest oppression, vomiting, nausea, a white, slimy tongue coating, and a wiry, slippery or soft, slippery pulse

Contraindications:

1. Do not use for dizziness and vertigo due to ascendant liver yang.
2. Do not use for dizziness and vertigo due to blood vacuity.

Formula explanation:

Within this formula, Pinellia dries dampness and transforms phlegm, downbears counterflow and stops vomiting. Gastrodia transforms phlegm and extinguishes wind. It also stops vertigo. These two used together are the essential medicinals for the treatment of wind phlegm dizziness, vertigo, and headache and are the two sovereign medicinals in this formula. Atractylodes is the minister. It fortifies the spleen and dries dampness. When combined with Pinellia and Gastrodia, these two's ability to dispel dampness, transform phlegm, and stop vertigo is boosted. Poria is an assistant. It fortifies the spleen and percolates dampness. Combined with Atractylodes, these two are able to treat phlegm at its root, *i.e.*, the spleen. Red Orange Peel, fresh Ginger, and Red Dates are also assistants. Red Orange Peel rectifies the qi and transforms phlegm. Fresh Ginger and Red Dates regulate and harmonize the spleen and stomach. Licorice is the messenger. It harmonizes the center and regulates the other medicinals.

Additions & subtractions:

For severe dizziness and vertigo, add Bombyx Batryticatus (*Jiang Can*) and bile(-treated) Rhizoma Arisaematis (*Dan Nan Xing*).

For frontal headache, add Radix Angelicae (*Bai Zhi*).

For severe headache, add Fructus Viticis (*Man Jing Zi*).

For indigestion due to food stagnation, add Fructus Crataegi (*Shan Zha*).

For abdominal pain and distention, add Fructus Amomi (*Sha Ren*) and Radix Saussureae Seu Vladimiriae (*Mu Xiang*).

For neck and shoulder tension, add Radix Puerariae Lobatae (*Ge Gen*).

For symptoms of hot phlegm, add Caulis In Taeniis Bambusae (*Zhu Ru*).

For concomitant qi vacuity, add Radix Panacis Ginseng (*Ren Shen*) and Radix Astragali Membranacei (*Huang Qi*).

For tubercular meningitis, add Buthus Martensis (*Quan Xie*), Lumbricus (*Di Long*), and Bombyx Batryticatus (*Jiang Can*).

For excessive accumulation of phlegm with headache or dizziness and weakness of the hands and feet, cold feet, sinusitis, and/or compulsive sleeping after meals, add Cortex Phellodendri (*Huang Bai*), Rhizoma Atractylodis (*Cang Zhu*), Radix Panacis Ginseng (*Ren Shen*), Radix Astragali Membranacei (*Huang Qi*), Rhizoma Alismatis (*Ze Xie*), Fructus Germinatus Hordei Vulgaris (*Mai Ya*), and Massa Medica

Fermentata (*Shen Qu*). This results in Li Dong-yuan's *Ban Xia Bai Zhu Tian Ma Tang* (Pinellia, Atractylodes, & Gastrodia Decoction).

For wind stroke with coma and lockjaw, first give *Su He Xiang Wan* (Liquid Styrax Pills) and then follow with this formula. In this case, subtract Licorice and Red Dates and add bile(-treated) Rhizoma Arisaematis (*Dan Nan Xing*) and Rhizoma Acori Graminei (*Shi Chang Pu*).

小柴胡湯和解供

半夏人參甘草從

更用黃芩和薑棗

少陽百病此為宗

Mnemonic verse for learning *Xiao Chai Hu Tang*

16

Xiao Shi Dao Zhi Ji
Dispersing Food, Conducting Stagnation Formulas

Formulas within this category disperse food stagnation. Food stagnation may be due to either lack of discipline and regularity in eating, liver qi stagnation, or spleen/stomach vacuity with loss of promotion of transportation and transformation. Because stagnant food is a yin accumulation which obstructs the free flow of yang qi, this obstruction to the flow of qi may give rise to transformative heat. However, if there is spleen vacuity or over-eating cold, raw foods, food stagnation may also be complicated by cold.

Representative formula: *Bao He Wan* (Protecting Harmony Pills)

Composition:

Fructus Crataegi (*Shan Zha*), 12g
Massa Medica Fermentata (*Shen Qu*), 9g
Rhizoma Pinelliae Ternatae (*Ban Xia*), 9g
Sclerotium Poriae Cocos (*Fu Ling*), 9g
Pericarpium Citri Reticulatae (*Chen Pi*), 6g
Fructus Forsythiae Suspensae (*Lian Qiao*), 9g
Semen Raphani Sativi (*Luo Bo Zi*), 12g

Functions: Disperses food and harmonizes the stomach

Indications: Food accumulation. Indigestion, diarrhea, abdominal pain, gastrointestinal flu, belching, acute exacerbation of chronic gastritis, hepatitis, acute pancreatitis, and acute or chronic cholecystitis.

Main signs & symptoms: Epigastric glomus, fullness, distention, and pain, acid eructations, nausea on eating, vomiting of undigested food, possible diarrhea, a foul mouth odor, a thick, slimy, possibly yellow tongue coating, and a slippery pulse

Contraindications:

1. Do not use unmodified in case of spleen vacuity.

Formula explanation:

Within this formula, Crataegus is the sovereign. It disperses food and drink accumulations and stagnation. In particular, it disperses accumulations of meat and greasy, slimy substances. Massa Medica Fermentata disperses food and fortifies the spleen. It also transforms alcohol and eliminates accumulations of rotten food. Radish Seeds precipitate the qi and disperse food and particularly disperse accumulation of grains. These are the minister medicinals in this prescription. When used together, these three medicinals disperse all types of accumulated and stagnant food stuffs. The assistants, Pinellia and Orange Peel, move the qi and transform stagnation, harmonize the stomach and stop vomiting. Poria fortifies the spleen and disinhibits dampness, harmonizes the center and stops diarrhea. Since food accumulations easily transform into heat, another assistant is added. Forsythia clears heat and scatters nodulation. When all these medicinals are combined together, food accumulation is transformed and the stomach qi is harmonized.

Additions & subtractions:

If food stagnation is severe, add Fructus Immaturus Citri Seu Ponciri (*Zhi Shi*) and Semen Arecae Catechu (*Bing Lang*).

Also if food stagnation and gastric distention are severe, add Fructus Immaturus Citri Seu Ponciri (*Zhi Shi*), Radix Saussureae Seu Vladimiriae (*Mu Xiang*), and Cortex Magnoliae Officinalis (*Hou Po*).

If the tongue coating is yellow, the pulse is rapid and there is bad breath, add Radix Scutellariae Baicalensis (*Huang Qin*) and Rhizoma Coptidis Chinensis (*Huang Lian*).

If there is constipation, add Radix Et Rhizoma Rhei (*Da Huang*) and Semen Arecae Catechu (*Bing Lang*).

For stomach flu, add Caulis Perillae Frutescentis (*Su Gen*) and Herba Agastachis Seu Pogostemi (*Huo Xiang*).

For food stagnation with spleen vacuity, add Rhizoma Atractylodis Macrocephalae (*Bai Zhu*). This results in *Da An Wan* (Great Quieting Pills).

For sweating on the head due to transformative heat, add Rhizoma Coptidis Chinensis (*Huang Lian*) fried in ginger juice.

For the initial stages of dysentery complicated by food stagnation, subtract Forsythia and Poria and add Rhizoma Coptidis Chinensis (*Huang Lian*), Semen Arecae Catechu (*Bing Lang*), and Fructus Immaturus Citri Seu Ponciri (*Zhi Shi*).

Also for dysentery with fever, vomiting, and diarrhea, add Rhizoma Coptidis Chinensis (*Huang Lian*), Radix Scutellariae Baicalensis (*Huang Qin*), and Radix Puerariae Lobatae (*Ge Gen*).

For disharmony of the liver and stomach with distention and pain in the chest and lateral costal regions and easy anger, add Radix Bupleuri (*Chai Hu*), Tuber Curcumae (*Yu Jin*), Rhizoma Cyperi Rotundi (*Xiang Fu*), and Radix Albus Paeoniae Lactiflorae (*Bai Shao*).

17

Sha Chong Ji
Killing Worms Formulas

In Chinese, the word *chong* means insect, worm, or bug. However, it also covers frogs, lizards, and snakes. Medically, it refers to parasites within the body. Most of these are species of worms. According to Chinese medical theory, worms arise in a damp, hot terrain. Typically, such damp heat is associated with spleen vacuity. If spleen vacuity is more severe, there may be accompanying coldness rather than heat, or both cold and heat.

General symptoms of worms include intermittent, periumbilical pain, gnawing hunger and the ability to eat even when there is abdominal pain, white spots on the cheeks, bruxism, vomiting of clear fluids, a peeled tongue coating, and a pulse which abruptly changes from large to small. Long-term parasitosis results in emaciation, fatigue, loss of appetite, poor vision and hearing, dry hair, and a large, distended abdomen.

Cautions & Contraindications:

1. For best effect, take worm-killing formulas on an empty stomach.
2. Do not use in the elderly or constitutionally weak.
3. Do not use during pregnancy.
4. After the parasites have been expelled, supplement the spleen and stomach to consolidate the treatment.

Representative formula: *Wu Mei Wan* (Mume Pills)

Composition:

Fructus Pruni Mume (*Wu Mei*), 15g
Herba Cum Radice Asari (*Xi Xin*), 3g
dry Rhizoma Zingiberis (*Gan Jiang*), 9g
Rhizoma Coptidis Chinensis (*Huang Lian*), 6g
Radix Angelicae Sinensis (*Dang Gui*), 9g
Radix Praeparatus Aconiti Carmichaeli (*Fu Zi*), 9g
Fructus Zanthoxyli Bungeani (*Shu Jiao*), 3g
Ramulus Cinnamomi (*Gui Zhi*), 9g
Radix Panacis Ginseng (*Ren Shen*), 9g
Cortex Phellodendri (*Huang Bo*), 9g

Functions: Warms the viscera and quiets roundworms

Indications: Roundworm inversion patterns. Ascariasis, biliary ascariasis, chronic dysentery, chronic gastritis, gastric ulcer, post-gastrectomy syndrome, neurosis, insomnia, and menstrual, premenstrual, and menopausal complaints associated with candidiasis and a combination of hot and cold, vacuity and repletion signs and symptoms, including endometriosis

Main signs & symptoms: Heart vexation, vomiting, sometimes have, sometimes stops, vomiting of food containing roundworms, inversion chill of the hands and feet, abdominal pain, possible prolonged dysentery or diarrhea, a peeled tongue coating, and hidden or wiry, tight pulse

Contraindications:

1. Do not use with explosive diarrhea.
2. Do not use with damp heat dysentery.

Formula explanation:

In this formula, heavy doses of Mume are used based on the ability of the sour flavor to control roundworms. Before being calmed, these were stirring and harassing. Zanthoxylum and Asarum are acrid flavored and are able to expel worms. Their nature is also warm, so they can warm the viscera and dispel cold. Coptis and Phellodendron are bitter and this bitterness is able to precipitate the roundworms. In addition, their coldness is able to clear heat above. The use of the above ingredients is based on the saying:

> When roundworms obtain (*i.e.*, encounter) sourness, they are calmed. When they obtain acridity, they subside. When they obtain bitter, they are able to be precipitated.

Additionally, Ginger, Cinnamon, and Aconite warm the viscera and dispel and precipitate cold. Ginseng and *Dang Gui* supplement and nourish the qi and blood. When combined with medicinals which warm the center, they boost the qi and warm the center at the same time as warming and supplementing lower burner vacuity cold, nourishing the blood and freeing the vessels, and regulating and harmonizing yin and yang. This then treats the inversion chilling of the four extremities.

Additions & subtractions:

To increase this formula's worm-killing and expelling functions, add Semen Quisqualis Indicae (*Shi Jun Zi*), Semen Arecae Catechu (*Bing Lang*), Cortex Radicis Meliae Azardachis (*Ku Lian Gen Pi*), and Semen Torreyae Grandis (*Fei Zi*).

In order to facilitate the excretion of parasites through the stools, add Radix Et Rhizoma Rhei (*Da Huang*).

For constipation, add Radix Et Rhizoma Rhei (*Da Huang*) and Semen Arecae Catechu (*Bing Lang*).

Also for constipation, add Fructus Immaturus Citri Seu Ponciri (*Zhi Shi*) and Semen Arecae Catechu (*Bing Lang*).

If there is no inversion chilling, subtract Cinnamon and Aconite.

If there is severe internal cold, subtract Phellodendron.

If there are no signs or symptoms of vacuity, subtract Ginseng and *Dang Gui*.

For severe abdominal pain, add Radix Saussureae Seu Vladimiriae (*Mu Xiang*) and Fructus Meliae Toosendan (*Chuan Lian Zi*).

For severe vomiting, add Fructus Evodiae Rutecarpae (*Wu Zhu Yu*) and Rhizoma Pinelliae Ternatae (*Ban Xia*).

For chronic, unremitting dysenteric diarrhea, subtract Ginseng and Phellodendron and replace Ramulus Cinnamomi with Cortex Cinnamomi (*Rou Gui*).

For chronic painful dysentery, add Radix Saussureae Seu Vladimiriae (*Mu Xiang*) and Radix Albus Paeoniae Lactiflorae (*Bai Shao*).

Chinese Bibliography _____

Chong Yong Fang Ji Jia Jian Chi (A Compilation of Additions & Subtractions for Commonly Used Formulas), Xu Hong-yen, New Medical Publishing Society, Taiwan, 1980

Fang Ji Xue (The Study of Formulas & Prescriptions), Guangzhou College of TCM, People's Medical Press, Beijing, 1983

Fang Ji Xue (The Study of Formulas & Prescriptions), Xu Ji-qun *et. al.*, Shanghai Science & Technology Press, Shanghai, 1986

Ying Hua Chong Yong Zhong Yi Chu Fang Shou Ce (An English-Chinese Handbook of Commonly Used TCM Formulas), Ou Ming, Joint Publishing Co., Ltd., Hong Kong, 1989

Zhong Yi Fang Ji Xue (The Study of TCM Formulas & Prescriptions), Fu Riu-qing, Hunan Science & Technology Press, Changsha, 1986

English Bibliography _____

Chinese Herbal Medicine: Formulas & Strategies, Bensky & Barolet, Eastland Press, Seattle, WA, 1990

A Clinical Guide to Chinese Herbs & Formulae, Chen & Li, Churchill Livingstone, UK, 1993

Commonly Used Chinese Herb Formulas with Illustrations, Hsu & Hsu, Oriental Healing Arts Institute, Los Angeles, CA, 1980

Handbook of Cinese Herbs & Formulas, Vol. II, Him-che Yeung, self-published, 1985

Herbal Formulas, Geng Jun-ying *et. al.*, New World Press, Beijing, 1991

Pearls from the Golden Cabinet, Subhuti Dharmananda, Oriental Healing Arts Institute, Long Beach, CA, 1988

Sixty-five Herbal Formulas for the California License Exam of Acupuncture, Chen & Chen, self-published, Garden Grove, CA, 1990

A Supplement to the Sixty-five Herbal Formulas for the California License Exam of Acupuncture, Chen & Chen, self-published, Garden Grove, CA, undated

Index

A

abdomen, dragging feeling in the lower 105
abdomen, pain in the 23
abdominal distention and pain 35, 157
abdominal distention, fullness, and pain 24
abdominal fullness, severe 27
abdominal glomus and fullness 38
abdominal masses, immobile subcostal 170
abdominal pain 6, 21, 23, 24, 26, 27, 35, 41, 42, 44, 45, 54, 56, 77, 78, 84, 87, 88, 92, 95, 100, 106, 107, 137, 143-145, 153, 160, 171, 172, 174, 232, 236, 239, 240, 242
abdominal pain, acute 23
abdominal pain and nausea, interior cold with 145
abdominal pain, cold 42, 153
abdominal pain due to cold stagnation 160
abdominal pain, lower 45, 106, 145
abdominal pain, postpartum 171
abdominal pain, severe 27, 42, 78, 174, 242
abdominal pain which likes both pressure and warmth 143
abortion, threatened 102, 108, 109
acidosis, tubular 146
acne 51, 69
acne rosacea 69
Addison's disease 115, 119
agalactia 99
albuminuria 119
aldosteronism, primary 146
amenorrhea 45, 106, 109, 124, 170, 171

anemia 47, 84, 94, 99, 106, 110-112, 115, 211
anemia, aplastic 111, 115
anemia, pernicious 99
anger, easy 52, 65, 94, 109, 169, 238
angina pectoris 84, 104, 137, 169-172
anus, burning heat around the 77
anxiety attacks 128
aphasia 179, 184, 187
appendicitis 23, 40
appetite, lack of, due to food stagnation 202
appetite, loss of 21, 36, 80, 96, 101, 159, 230, 239
appetite, reduced 47, 49, 221
apraxia 184, 187
arteriosclerosis, cerebral 99, 184, 186
arthritis 4, 5, 9, 88-90, 119, 205, 211, 213, 214
arthritis of the upper extremities 9
arthritis, rheumatoid 4, 89, 90, 205, 211, 213
ascariasis, biliary 40, 44, 240
ascites 28, 207, 228
ascites due to cirrhosis 28
asthma 4, 119, 122, 161, 211, 228
asthma, bronchial 119, 211, 228
asthma, cardiac 228
asthma, chronic bronchial 119
asthma, severe 122
asthma with palpitations and dizziness 122
auditory canal, boils and carbuncles in the vestibular and external 74

B

Basedow's disease 211
bed-wetting, pediatric 104
belching 155, 157, 184, 212, 236

H

W

Y

Index

OTHER BOOKS ON CHINESE MEDICINE AVAILABLE FROM BLUE POPPY PRESS

1775 Linden Ave ○ Boulder, CO 80304
For ordering 1-800-487-9296
PH. 303\447-8372 FAX 303\447-0740

THE HEART & ESSENCE Of Dan-xi's Methods of Treatment by Zhu Dan-xi, trans. by Yang Shou-zhong. ISBN 0-936185-50-3, $24.95

HOW TO WRITE A TCM HERBAL FORMULA A Logical Methodology for the Formulation & Administration of Chinese Herbal Medicine in Decoction, by Bob Flaws, ISBN 0-936185-49-X, $10.95

FULFILLING THE ESSENCE: A Handbook of Traditional & Contemporary Chinese Treatments for Female Infertility by Bob Flaws. ISBN 0-936185-48-1, $19.95

STATEMENTS OF FACT IN TRADITIONAL CHINESE MEDICINE by Bob Flaws. ISBN 0-936185-52-X, $10.95

IMPERIAL SECRETS OF HEALTH & LONGEVITY by Bob Flaws, ISBN 0-936185-51-1, $9.95

THE MEDICAL I CHING: Oracle of the Healer Within by Miki Shima, OMD, ISBN 0-936185-38-4, $19.95

THE SYSTEMATIC CLASSIC OF ACUPUNCTURE /MOXIBUSTION by Huang-fu Mi, trans. by Yang Shou-zhong and Charles Chace, ISBN 0-936185-29-5, hardback edition, $79.95

CHINESE PEDIATRIC MASSAGE THERAPY A Parent's & Practitioner's Guide to the Treatment and Prevention of Childhood Disease, by Fan Ya-li. ISBN 0-936185-54-6, $12.95

RECENT TCM RESEARCH FROM CHINA trans. by Bob Flaws & Charles Chace. ISBN 0-936185-56-2, $18.95

PMS: Its Cause, Diagnosis & Treatment According to Traditional Chinese Medicine by Bob Flaws ISBN 0-936185-22-8 $16.95

EXTRA TREATISES BASED ON INVESTIGATION & INQUIRY: A Translation of Zhu Dan-xi's *Ge Zhi Yu Lun*, trans. by Yang Shou-zhong & Duan Wu-jin, ISBN 0-936185-53-8, $15.95

THE DIVINELY
RESPONDING CLASSIC: A
Translation of the *Shen Ying
Jing* by Yang Shou-zhong and
Liu Feng-ting, ISBN 0-936185-
55-4, $18.95

A NEW AMERICAN
ACUPUNCTURE:
Acupuncture Osteopathy, by Mark
Seem, ISBN 0-936185-44-9,
$19.95

SCATOLOGY & THE
GATE OF LIFE: The Role
of the Large Intestine in
Immunity, An Integrated
Chinese-Western Approach
by Bob Flaws ISBN 0-936185-20-
1 $14.95

MENOPAUSE, A Second
Spring: Making A Smooth
Transition with Traditional
Chinese Medicine by Honora
Lee Wolfe ISBN 0-936185-18-X
$14.95

MIGRAINES &
TRADITIONAL CHINESE
MEDICINE: A Layperson's
Guide by Bob Flaws ISBN 0-
936185-15-5 $11.95

STICKING TO THE
POINT: A Rational
Methodology for the Step by
Step Administration of an
Acupuncture Treatment by
Bob Flaws ISBN 0-936185-17-1
$16.95

ENDOMETRIOSIS &
INFERTILITY AND
TRADITIONAL CHINESE
MEDICINE: A Laywoman's
Guide by Bob Flaws ISBN 0-
936185-14-7 $9.95

THE BREAST
CONNECTION: A
Laywoman's Guide to the
Treatment of Breast Disease
by Chinese Medicine
by Honora Lee Wolfe ISBN 0-
936185-61-9 $9.95

NINE OUNCES: A Nine Part
Program For The Prevention
of AIDS in HIV Positive
Persons by Bob Flaws ISBN 0-
936185-12-0 $9.95

THE TREATMENT OF
CANCER BY
INTEGRATED
CHINESE-WESTERN
MEDICINE by Zhang Dai-
zhao, trans. by Zhang Ting-liang
ISBN 0-936185-11-2 $18.95

A HANDBOOK OF
TRADITIONAL CHINESE
DERMATOLOGY by Liang
Jian-hui, trans. by Zhang Ting-
liang & Bob Flaws, ISBN 0-
936185-07-4 $15.95

A HANDBOOK OF
TRADITIONAL CHINESE
GYNECOLOGY by Zhejiang
College of TCM, trans. by Zhang
Ting-liang, ISBN 0-936185-06-6
(2nd edit.) $21.95

PRINCE WEN HUI'S COOK: Chinese Dietary Therapy by Bob Flaws & Honora Lee Wolfe, ISBN 0-912111-05-4, $12.95 (Published by Paradigm Press, Brookline, MA)

THE DAO OF INCREASING LONGEVITY AND CONSERVING ONE'S LIFE by Anna Lin & Bob Flaws, ISBN 0-936185-24-4 $16.95

FIRE IN THE VALLEY: The TCM Diagnosis and Treatment of Vaginal Diseases by Bob Flaws ISBN 0-936185-25-2 $16.95

HIGHLIGHTS OF ANCIENT ACUPUNCTURE PRESCRIPTIONS trans. by Honora Lee Wolfe & Rose Crescenz ISBN 0-936185-23-6 $14.95

ARISAL OF THE CLEAR: A Simple Guide to Healthy Eating According to Traditional Chinese Medicine by Bob Flaws, ISBN #-936185-27-9 $8.95

PEDIATRIC BRONCHITIS: ITS CAUSE, DIAGNOSIS & TREATMENT ACCORDING TO TRADITIONAL CHINESE MEDICINE trans. by Gao Yu-li and Bob Flaws, ISBN 0-936185-26-0 $15.95

AIDS & ITS TREATMENT ACCORDING TO TRADITIONAL CHINESE MEDICINE by Huang Bing-shan, trans. by Fu-Di & Bob Flaws, ISBN 0-936185-28-7 $24.95

ACUTE ABDOMINAL SYNDROMES: Their Diagnosis & Treatment by Combined Chinese-Western Medicine by Alon Marcus, ISBN 0-936185-31-7 $16.95

MY SISTER, THE MOON: The Diagnosis & Treatment of Menstrual Diseases by Traditional Chinese Medicine by Bob Flaws, ISBN 0-936185-34-1, $24.95

FU QING-ZHU'S GYNECOLOGY trans. by Yang Shou-zhong and Liu Da-wei, ISBN 0-936185-35-X, $21.95

FLESHING OUT THE BONES: The Importance of Case Histories in Chinese Medicine by Charles Chace. ISBN 0-936185-30-9, $18.95

CLASSICAL MOXIBUSTION SKILLS IN CONTEMPORARY CLINICAL PRACTICE by Sung Baek, ISBN 0-936185-16-3 $10.95

MASTER TONG'S ACUPUNCTURE: An Ancient Lineage for Modern Practice, trans. and commentary by Miriam Lee, OMD, ISBN 0-936185-37-6, $19.95

A HANDBOOK OF TCM UROLOGY & MALE SEXUAL DYSFUNCTION by Anna Lin, OMD, ISBN 0-936185-36-8, $16.95

Li Dong-yuan's TREATISE ON THE SPLEEN & STOMACH, A Translation of the *Pi Wei Lun* by Yang Shou-zhong & Li Jian-yong, ISBN 0-936185-41-4, $21.95

PATH OF PREGNANCY, VOL. I, Gestational Disorders by Bob Flaws, ISBN 0-936185-39-2, $16.95

PATH OF PREGNANCY, VOL. II, Postpartum Diseases by Bob Flaws, ISBN 0-936185-42-2, $18.95

How to Have a HEALTHY PREGNANCY, HEALTHY BIRTH with Traditional Chinese Medicine by Honora Lee Wolfe, ISBN 0-936185-40-6, $9.95

MASTER HUA'S CLASSIC OF THE CENTRAL VISCERA by Hua Tuo, translated by Yang Shou-zhong, ISBN 0-936185-43-0, $21.95

SEVENTY ESSENTIAL TCM FORMULAS FOR BEGINNERS by Bob Flaws, ISBN 0-936185-59-7, $19.95

CHINESE MEDICINAL WINES by Bob Flaws, ISBN 0-936185-58-9, $18.95

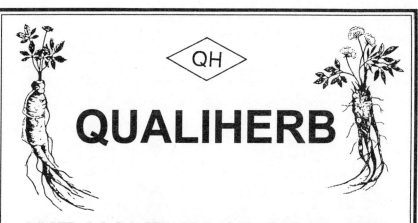